LOW FODMAP

DIET

All You Need to Know About It's Diagnosis & Treatment

(Low Fodmap Diet Cookbook for Gut Health)

Paula Silva

Published by Alex Howard

Low Fodmap Diet: All You Need to Know About It's Diagnosis & Treatment
(Low Fodmap Diet Cookbook for Gut Health)

ISBN 978-1-990169-20-5

Legal & Disclaimer

The information contained in this book is not designed to replace or take the place of any form of medicine or professional medical advice. The information in this book has been provided for educational and entertainment purposes only.

Table of contents

Part 1

Introduction

If you have ever found yourself running to the convenience after eating certain foods or trying hard to hold in gas so as not to make the human race extinct, if this is accompanied by abdominal discomfort, a change in form or frequency of your stool (i.e if you get diarrhoea or constipation), if you even feel pain while stooling and you find that these happen at least once a week for three to six months, then you probably have IBS (**Irritable Bowel Syndrome**).

Don't be alarmed, you aren't going to have to drag your entrails around or something, while IBS can be quite uncomfortable for you and the people around you, I am sure you will be glad to hear that it isn't life threatening at all.

So, I am about to bring something big into play here, **FODMAPs**. No, they are not another medical condition, but more often than not, they are responsible for IBS. Now I can see that you are interested, so let's get right into it.

So, who exactly are these bad guys? FODMAPs are short for **"Fermentable Oligo, Di-, Monosaccharides And Polyols"**. I know it is a bit of a mouthful but it simply refers to a group of short chain carbs that are not well absorbed by the body which results in bloating, flatulence, diarrhoea, abdominal pain etc.

Now that you know the culprit, the logical response would be to cut back on high-FODMAP foods right? Right! That's where the low-FODMAP diet comes in. Do not be fooled by the word "diet" cozily seating in there, it is not a weight loss diet, all it does is relieve the symptoms of IBS.

I can see that you are practically dancing in your shoes, finally a solution! But I am going to have to put a teeny weeny smudge on that by informing you that the low-FODMAP diet doesn't work for everyone. It works for at least four out of five people, that is a good figure right? So, who is to say it won't work for you? There is no harm in trying. The problem is, when you have IBS, knowing what to eat can be hard, because you will always wonder if it will upset your stomach, that is why I'd say this book is exactly what you need, together we will make mouth watering recipes that will help relieve your symptoms.

But before all that, I'd like for us to delve deeper into the relationship between FODMAPs and IBS. Are you ready? Let's jump right in!

Chapter One: Irritable Bowel Syndrome

IBS (**Irritable Bowel Syndrome**) is a chronic long-term gastrointestinal condition that causes recurrent constipation or diarrhoea, abdominal pain, bloating and flatulence, it is most often caused by anxiety, stress, depression, the kind of food consumed by the individual or a past history of intestinal infection.

It is surprisingly very common even though many people do not know they have it until they are diagnosed.

It is also referred to as nervous colon, spastic colitis, and mucous colitis, just a couple of fancy names for a very uncomfortable condition. Most times, the biggest fear many people have is of the condition getting worse over time. Honestly, in some cases it does and in some others, it doesn't. It just depends on the method used to manage the condition. The symptoms will usually continue if nothing is done and I am sure you can guess how difficult that would be. The only bright spot in this cloud of gloom is the fact that this condition doesn't progress into something more serious and life threatening like cancer, ulcerative colitis or bleeding.

Symptoms

If you are very observant, you won't need a genie to tell you that you have IBS, the symptoms are pretty simple to identify, but just to be on the safe side, the most common symptoms to look out for are;

1. Bloating or swelling of the stomach.
2. Cramping or abdominal discomfort
3. Change in your bowel habit.
4. A sudden need to use the toilet (e.g in the middle of a meal)
5. Passing of mucus when stooling.
6. Flatulence

7. The need to pass stool even after doing so.

These symptoms might get worse after meals and may last for several days before they subside or get completely resolved.

Because of the individuality of every being, they are each affected differently, some may feel worse than others and have their symptoms resolve themselves over a short period of time, while others might feel small recurrent discomforts that may persist over a longer period of time and as such, symptoms may also vary from person to person. Below are a few uncommon symptoms related to the condition.

1. Irregular Menstruation
2. Migraines or Headaches
3. Bouts of tiredness or fatigue
4. Pain during of after intercourse for females
5. Muscle or joint pain
6. Frequent urination
7. Bad breath
8. Dehydration
9. Shame, depression or anxiety, especially due to the embarrassment that accompany the condition.

Triggers

Triggers are those little things that make your IBS symptoms worse or flare up after a short period of dormancy. Like I said earlier, you'd have to be really observant for things like these because it might be hard to pinpoint the exact thing that triggered your symptoms, especially if your symptoms start after a while, it's not like you keep a log book of every single thing that passes through your mouth. The logical solution will be to avoid well known triggers of IBS, then wait to see how that works for you. When you figure out what your triggers are, then you can keep your bloating, diarrhoea, constipation and abdominal pain under control. There are a few things that a notorious for triggering IBS and they are;

Anxiety/Stress

At one point or the other, I am sure we have all been in situations where we were anxious about something, maybe a presentation, job or a meeting. In cases like that, some people get sick to their stomachs. The same can happen to people with IBS, their symptoms might be triggered after a long day at work, before an exam etc. As we all know, anxiety and stress is completely unavoidable, it is not something that is premeditated, it just happens, so the question is, how do you deal with this if you can't avoid it? Well, you can manage it. So, below are a few tips to help you manage your anxiety and stress;

1. Have some fun! You don't always have to be Mr.Scrooge, always grumpy and serious. Sometimes you just have to loosen up a bit, sing, dance, make friends and smile, it helps ease stress and lightens your mood.
2. Choose a healthy lifestyle; get enough sleep so that you do not look like a red eyed monster every morning, exercise regularly (even if it's a few rounds around your house every morning), eat recommended foods that work for your IBS.
3. Confide in friends or family; It really helps to have people around who understand what you are going through and empathize with you, it makes you feel less self-conscious and reduces anxiety.
4. Therapy; This might seem totally cliche, but behavioral therapy is guaranteed to help you feel with stress and anxiety, you could also try hypnotherapy, relaxation therapy, psychotherapy or cognitive psychotherapy.

Menstruation

I am sorry to be the bearer of bad news, but symptoms of IBS tend to get worse when women are on their periods. Sadly, there isn't much that can be done to prevent it, but there are a few tips that are sure to ease the discomfort at that time of the month.

1. You can meet a doctor for prescriptions to help treat severe PMS.
2. Use contraceptive pills to make your period regular and help reduce dysmenorrhea, but be careful because they can have side effects like cramps, nausea, bloating etc.

Diet

Individual diet plays a huge role in IBS, what you eat can affect you positively or negatively. If you notice that your symptoms worsen or improve anytime you eat something, then you are probably triggered by it. Things like milk, alcohol or chocolate may make you have diarrhoea or constipation. Even vegetables, sodas and fruits can trigger abdominal discomfort and bloating.

Common foods that trigger bloating or abdominal discomfort are;

- Bagels
- Celery
- Carrots
- Beans
- Prunes
- Raisins
- Onions
- Bananas
- Pretzels
- Brussels sprouts

Diets That trigger IBS-Related Diarrhoea

If you have IBS, listed below are a few foods that tend to make IBS-related diarrhoea worse:

1. Dairy products, especially for people who are lactose intolerant.
2. Carbonated drinks. If you find yourself walking towards the vending machine at every given chance, then you might consider putting a stop to it.
3. Fried or fatty foods. I know how absolutely tempting those road side foods are, with the aromas wafting into your

nostrils, beckoning you and eventually leading to abdominal discomfort. So next time you find yourself walking towards that fast-food stand, ask yourself, is it worth it? Is it worth the endless trips to the toilet, if not, then I guess you have your answer.

4. Drinks or foods that contain sorbitol, chocolate, fructose, caffeine, or alcohol.
5. Eating very large meals. So I guess you might reconsider eating till you burst your seams this weekend.
6. Foods that contain gluten e.g. wheat, especially to those who are allergic to it.
7. Consuming too much fiber, especially those that are insoluble, like vegetables or the skin of some fruits.

Now that you know what to avoid so as to not worsen your IBS-related diarrhoea, here are a few tips to help you manage it;

1. Do not drink water while eating, you could try drinking it an hour before or after your meal.
2. Avoid gassy foods like celery, beans, wheat, and brussels sprouts, they tend to cause gas and bloating, which would make your diarrhoea worse.
3. Try to have soluble fibers in moderate amounts. So you could try some brown rice, dried fruits, whole wheat breads, whole-grain pasta, barley and oats, they add bulk to your stool.
4. Eat smaller portions of cabbage, broccoli and onions, they cause gas which will eventually worsen your diarrhoea.
5. See a dietician concerning any diet related allergies you might have.
6. Try not to eat food at opposite temperatures, you should try until they are almost the same temperature i.e you shouldn't eat steaming hot food with another that is totally cold. In a case like this, you could put the cold one in the microwave until it is heated and close to the temperature of the hot food, if not, heat them both and allow them to cool until they are both warm.

Diets That Trigger IBS-Related Constipation

Just as some foods will have you dashing for the nearest convenience, some will have you begging the heavens for a chance to relieve your bowels, all to no avail. So, listed below are a few common triggers for IBS-related constipation;

- High-protein diets
- Cereals or breads made with refined grains
- Dairy products like cheese
- High-carb processed foods like cookies or chips.
- Alcohol, coffee and carbonated drinks.

Here are a few tips to help you manage your IBS-related constipation;

1. Stay hydrated; it is even medically recommended that you drink about two litres of water per day. I know you won't be able to drink it all in one go, except you have the world's largest bladder of course.
2. Slowly increase your fiber intake to about 3 grams daily until your are consuming at least 38 grams(for men) and 25 grams (for women). You can get your desired amount from vegetables, fruits, beans and cereals.
3. Reduce your intake of sugar rich foods. As it stands, you'll have to cut back on your favorite beverages, no matter how difficult it may seem.
4. A small amount of flaxseed, sprinkled over vegetables or salad can work wonders.

Medication

I am pretty sure that you must have noticed that some drugs have side effects, which are boldly written in those little pieces of paper you find in the pack, and these side effects may trigger diarrhoea or constipation. A few of the common culprits in this case are;

- Antidepressants (not all of them)
- Antibiotics
- Drugs that contain sorbitol (e.g cough syrups)

These drug related triggers can be managed by;

1. Use only prescribed antidepressants, and use them as instructed.
2. Talk to a professional about any drug you want to take before using it.

Other triggers may include;

1. Irregular exercise.
2. Eating too much too fast.
3. Eating while laying down or driving.
4. Chewing gum.

How to manage it;

1. Eat while sitting
2. Try to exercise regularly
3. Talk to your doctor for options on drugs that are safe to take in your condition

Causes Of Ibs

No particular cause has been found till date, but it is medically proven not to be life-threatening, contagious or cancerous. But there are a few factors that may contribute to the development of IBS, and they are;

- Hormones
- An individual's mental or emotional state (e.g people with PTSD stand a higher chance of getting IBS)
- An irregularity in the function of the digestive system
- Diet
- Stress
- High sensitivity to pain of the digestive organs
- An inability to fight infections

Is Ibs Curable?

Unfortunately, there has been no cure found for IBS, but that doesn't mean you'll have to live in discomfort for the rest of your life, all it takes is a change of habits, a good doctor, a few new recipes and you are good to go. Since the cure for IBS hasn't yet been found, treatment aims to improve the quality of life by relieving symptoms.

Treatment

As i mentioned above, treatment of IBS is aimed at relieving symptoms and flares, it mostly involves a change in diet, reducing stress and a couple of lifestyle changes.

Here are a few tips to go by;

1. Try not to skip meals.
2. Reduce your intake of alcohol.
3. Reduce your intake of certain vegetables and fruits.
4. Eating at about the same time each day.
5. Try to eat slowly.
6. Stay hydrated.
7. Avoid foods or products that contain sugar alternatives.
8. Eat gluten free foods.
9. Avoid sugary and carbonated beverages.
10. Go for oat-based foods.

Treatment Of Stress-Related IBS

1. Practice a few relaxation techniques like yoga, meditation, Tai chi. You could even try exercising of it relaxes you.
2. Cognitive Behavioral therapy or stress counselling.

Now that we know basically everything there is to know about IBS, I think it's high time we also look at FODMAPs, these little devils.

Chapter Two: What Are The Fodmaps

I am sure you can remember how much of a mouthful this word is, so let's start by breaking them down into smaller more understandable pieces.

F-ermentable: This word refers to short chain carbohydrates that can not be absorbed by the body, so what these little monsters do is to travel through the digestive tract and stop at the small intestines, where they hold small parties with gut bacteria and get fermented in the process, which results in the production of gas as a byproduct. So next time you pass wind, think about these little villains—fermentables.

O-ligosaccharides: Wherever you see the word "saccharide" just have it in mind that it's just a fancy word for "sugar". Of Course you can't bandy such a big word at breakfast but I am sure it will be useful to you sometime, while the word "Oligo" means few in greek. So if you were to put the two words side by side, it would literally translate to "few sugars" which basically means small sugars. Examples of foods that contain oligosaccharides are beans, onions, rye, lentils, wheat, and garlic.

D-isaccharides: As you might have already guessed, the prefix "Di" means two, put together with "saccharides" it means two sugars or double sugars. It refers to those carbohydrates that are composed of two monosaccharides. Examples are maltose, lactose and sucrose which are found in foods like yoghurts, soft cheeses and milk.

M-onosaccharides: This refers to the simplest type of sugar there is. Infact, most sugars (e.g disaccharides) are built from it. The word "mono" means one and from that you can tell that it is composed of a single sugar molecule and cannot be further broken down. An example of monosaccharides is fructose, which can be found in foods like apples, honey and many other fruits.

P-olyols: This refers to a group of organic compounds that have several hydroxyl groups. Most of them are naturally occurring in some fruits like avocados, peaches, pears and cherries.

There are a class of polyols called sugar alcohols, they are non-nutritive sweeteners and are mostly found in diabetic or low carb products and chewing gum. Examples of polyols are isomalt and xylitol.

High-Fodmap Foods

Written below is a list of High-FODMAP foods, but note that the list is not exhaustive, due to the difference in the methods used to process foods in different countries, as well as the different additives used.

Foods Containing Excess Fructose

1. Sugars: High fructose corn syrup, honey etc.
2. Vegetables: Peas, artichokes, asparagus etc.
3. Fruits: Tinned fruits preserved in their natural juice, apples, dried fruits, pears, mangoes, cherries etc.

Fructans (Galacto-oligosaccharides and Fructo-oligosaccharides)

1. Fiber: Inulin
2. Legumes and Fruits: Red kidney beans, persimmon, garlic, lentils, onions, beans, peaches, artichokes, watermelon etc.
3. Grain: couscous, rye and rye products, pasta, wheat and wheat products.

Polyols-Mannitol

1. Fruits: watermelon
2. Vegetables: peas, mushrooms, cauliflower, etc.

Polyols- Sorbitol

1. Beverages: pear and apple juice, etc.
2. Fruits: plums, blackberries, apples, nectarines, pears, apricots.

Polyols-Mannitol And Sorbitol

1. Sweetener: maltitol, sugar free gums, chocolates and hard candies containing sorbitol, isomalt, mannitol, etc.

Lactose

1. Dairy products: Ice cream, soft cheeses, custard etc.
2. Yoghurts and milk: Yoghurts and low fat milk.

Please note that this list is not definitive, you might not have a problem with any of the foods listed above, but you might for something else. It only depends on your system, what might trigger your friends symptoms might not disturb you.

Are Fodmaps Bad For You?

I am sure you must have raised a brow when you noticed that foods like avocados, peas, lentils, even apples were being brandished as bad guys and forced into orange overalls and made to take mug shots, but the question is, are they really bad for you? Well, they are all naturally healthy!

A bit confused? Let's just say these little fellas aren't really responsible, or can you be made responsible for what you are made of? In this case it's the short chain carbohydrates that these foods contain that we have a problem with, so should we be blamed? After all we are the ones unable to properly break them down. So what exactly does this mean? It means these little divas travel through your digestive system without a single hair out of place, and since they remain unchanged due to your inability to break them down, they make their presence known by drawing fluid into the bowel, and as you might have guessed, results in nothing but discomfort for you.

Chapter Three: The Role Of Fodmaps In Digestive Problems

We are all different from each other, and as such, our digestive systems are highly different. Over time, our reactions to some foods will change, it could be due to age, the overall health of one's digestive system, environment or lifestyle. You might notice that you have no problem with certain foods in your youth, but as you age, you will notice that you become more intolerant. Sometimes, you might not even have a problem with a certain food today, but it may cause you extreme discomfort the next day. Noone till date knows why this dramatic changes occur because the human digestive system is very complex. I am sure that you didn't know that your digestive tract has up to a hundred nerve endings, that's even more than that of your spine! Amazing right? If you ask me, I'd say we've barely scratched the surface where the digestive system is concerned. I mean, how can we claim to fully understand something so amazingly complex?

It might sound a little bit gross but I am sure you didn't know that your lower digestive tract is home to many bacteria, both good and bad, and there is a definite cycle in motion on the microbial level. When you are stressed or Ill, the medicines you take all affect your gut bacteria, because they feed off of what you eat.

Unfortunately, as I have mentioned severally before, we are unable to produce the enzymes that are needed to breakdown FODMAPs, and they eventually travel through the small intestine and into the large intestine.

But if you find yourself frequently dealing with digestive problems, maybe chronic gas, constipation, diarrhoea, bloating and abdominal (which are all symptoms of IBS), then you are probably sensitive to high-FODMAP foods.

How Fodmaps Affect The Gut

When FODMAPs are introduced into the digestive system, they increase the production of intestinal gas and cause fluid changes. Small FODMAP molecules, exert an osmotic effect in the intestines which is the reason why fluids are drawn into the bowels, and gut bacteria waste no time working on FODMAPs which causes them to ferment and produce gas and as a result, the bowels get distended, which is why you tend to get bloated or have abdominal pain. It also alters the way the muscles of the bowels contract. When peristalsis (forward movement) is increased, it can cause diarrhoea for some and constipation in others. For example, fructose can draw twice as much fluids into your bowels than glucose(which is not a FODMAP) because it is "osmotically active" .

A lot of people are of the misconception that the inability to break down FODMAPS happens in only people with IBS, which is a very wrong assumption because even perfectly healthy people find it difficult to breakdown FODMAPs, which is perfectly normal. Although, it is only in people with IBS that symptoms are easily triggered, which may be as a result of;

1. The type of bacteria in the bowels; when there is an overgrowth of bacteria in the small intestine, it results in a condition called "**SIBO**" or "small intestine bacterial overgrowth" which leads to excessive gas production in the bowels, which as you know, results in bloating, abdominal pain, distension etc.
2. The manner in which the muscles of the bowels respond to distension; this may result in fast or slow passage of stool in the bowels. The gut is really sensitive, so it easily picks up on changes or any alterations in the gut environment and interacts with the immune system and nervous system in response to these changes. Which means people with IBS

have lower pain tolerance when their bowels are distended than healthy adults.

These two factors are what determine a person's reaction to FODMAPs, but there are those who aren't sensitive to FODMAPs, so they won't react the same way a person with IBS will, even with the factors listed above. This is thought to be as a result of a condition called colonic hypersensitivity, which is pretty common in people with IBS. So it's not like there is anything special about those who do not have colonic hypersensitivity, they are just lucky! Because these we are all unable to breakdown these short-chain carbs, they just bother the unlucky ones. But the question is why? Like i said before, it's mostly due to a person's hypersensitivity to certain changes to the gut environment, certain illnesses or stress.

Chapter Four: How To Practice The Low Fodmap Diet

The low-FODMAP diet aims to remove or reduce foods that are high in FODMAPs from our diet, but it can be a little tricky because there isn't any sure way of measuring the amount of FODMAPs found in foods. Although, it's not impossible. A group of researchers at Monash University in Melbourne, Australia, were the first to conduct a research to observe if a low-FODMAP diet would help relieve the symptoms of IBS and even went further to measure the FODMAP content of a lot of foods through food analysis. Since it's being recommended as a way to manage IBS, I would say that research was a success.

A lot of people would assume that the low-FODMAP diet is like every other diet out there, aim at helping people manage and lose weight, it isn't. It's sole aim is to help people eliminate foods that are high in short-chain carbs from their diet, as a way to reduce recurrent symptoms of IBS. But before jumping head first into the diet as it may seem like a heaven sent solution to your problem, I would advise you to have a chat with your doctor or dietician about it first because the diet is very restrictive.

Who Should You Talk to About The Diet?

If you are interested in starting the low-FODMAP diet, you need the approval of a registered dietician, who can advise you on which foods to avoid or eat and help you as you eliminate and reintroduce new foods into your diet until you figure out those that trigger you. You also need a dietician because you need to know how long to stay on the diet as it isn't a long term plan, it is only recommended for at least 2-6 weeks at a time, at which point you must already have figured out the foods that trigger you and avoid them.

Possible Side Effects Of The Diet

Because the restrictions placed on the low-FODMAP diet, you will need to discuss with your dietician so he can help you formulate a dietary plan to make up for the nutrients you will be eliminating from your diet. You may need to take a couple of mineral and vitamin supplements.

How Does It Work?

The low-FODMAP diet has three phases;

- **Elimination Phase**: This period refers to the first 3-8 weeks of the diet, where a person is required to cut back on all foods with high FODMAP content.
- **Reintroduction**: This period begins immediately after the elimination phase, it requires the individual to slowly reintroduce FODMAPs into their diet, one at a time, about every 3-7 days, then observe and see which foods trigger their symptoms.
- **Maintenance**: This is the simplest part of the low-FODMAP diet, as it only requires you to try to maintain a normal diet, by limiting the amount of FODMAPs you consume. Some might even be able to revert back to their previous eating pattern, eating some or all type of FODMAPs without any symptoms, while others will do perfectly fine as far as they avoid the foods that trigger them.

Is The Low-FODMAP Diet For Me?

First of all, you need to be certain that what you have is IBS. So, the first step would be to get yourself checked up by a certified doctor because it easy to mistaken your systems for something relating to celiac disease, inflammatory bowel diseases or bowel cancer.

Also, not all IBS symptoms are caused or triggered by high-FODMAP foods, some are triggered by spicy, high fat foods or caffeine. Your dietician would recommend an alternative form of treatment if your symptoms are not triggered by high-FODMAP foods since the low-FODMAP diet might not be suitable for you.

Advantages

The first thing you need to bear in mind is that the low-FODMAP diet isn't the solution to every single digestive problem there is out there, and it is not a quick weight loss plan. However, it has shown to completely change the lives of people with IBS for the better. Although it is really hard to keep up with because of its restrictions, the upsides make it totally worth it. So, listed below are a few advantages;

1. Helps you identify triggers; People who have allergic reactions to certain things go to great lengths to avoid them, it's the same for the low-FODMAP diet, it helps you identify those foods that you need to avoid. The diet is even referred to as a diagnostic treatment by some experts because of the reintroduction phase which helps you identify those foods that are most likely to set you off.
2. Alleviates symptoms of IBS: This is one of the biggest and most important role of the low-FODMAP diet. Infact, most of the research done on the diet has a lot to do with treating IBS symptoms. At least 76% of patients diagnosed with IBS reported a marked improvement when they began the low-FODMAP diet.
3. Founded by professionals: If you fear that the idea of the low-FODMAP diet is still novel, then you have no cause to worry because it was highly researched and founded by certified professionals. The research team at Monash University in Melbourne, Australia, are highly trained.The university has had several groundbreaking findings and is Australia's largest. The hypothesis that was published in 2005 was led by Susan Shepherd and Peter Gibson. They were of the opinion that FODMAPs increases one's chances of getting crohn's disease, as they advanced in their studies, it became clear that the low-FODMAP diet was better suited

for treating IBS. Over time, more researchers studied the diet and it's benefits.

4. Reduces inflammation in patients with IBD: There is currently no cure for some IB (irritable bowel) diseases like Crohn's disease and ulcerative colitis, but the low-FODMAP diet has proven to have positive effects on patients with IBD. Although the low-FODMAP diet has proven very helpful to many people, it is not guaranteed to work for everyone.

Disadvantages

Although the diet improves your digestive health, it isn't easy to follow. Going on dates or family dinners or gatherings can be very challenging because you will have to be very selective of what you eat. You can be sure of naturally cooked foods, but what of additives? I am pretty sure you get the picture. It can't always be rosy, right? So, listed below are a few downsides associated to the diet;

1. It is not a long-term solution; most times when we are diagnosed with a condition, the first thing that comes to mind is "how do I get rid of it?", but sometimes it's not that easy. In this case, the low-FODMAP diet isn't a long-term treatment plan and it doesn't cure all digestive problems. As mentioned above, it only aims at improving the quality of life of people with IBS and help them manage the condition. But if done right, you can get quick relief. The elimination phase lasts only a few weeks, but a lot of people start to have fewer symptoms and feel better at this point, but once this phase is over, some people might get some of all of their symptoms back, that's why you need the reintroduction phase to pinpoint your triggers. It might be a bit tempting to maintain the diet even after the expected timeline. I mean, who doesn't want to feel better. But experts suggest that you limit your intake of high-FODMAP foods instead of eliminating them completely so as not to develop a dietary deficiency.

2. Not recommended for children and pregnant women; It is natural for pregnant women to suffer from a few digestive problems like constipation, some would immediately go on a low-FODMAP diet as a way to tackle the problem, but it is not recommended because the foetus needs various nutrients to grow properly. Children are also discouraged from going on the low-FODMAP diet as they have many nutritional needs. There hasn't been sufficient research as of yet to ascertain the safety of the diet for pregnant women and children.

3. It has too many restrictions; This is the reason why the low-FODMAP diet isn't recommended as a long-term plan. That is why you are advised to start the diet under the guidance of a certified dietician because there is always going to be a concern for your nutritional needs to be met. FODMAPs are also encouraged in small amounts as they are beneficial to the growth of good bacteria in the gut. So, you can't go on a FODMAP free diet indefinitely, as some point or the other, your body is going to rebel with pitchforks and burning torches until you give them what they need.

4. Vegetarians/Vegans; The vegetarian/vegan diet is already restrictive on its own, so those who want to try the low-FODMAP diet are advised to find an alternative source for their protein oats, seeds, tempeh, quinoa, tofu etc.

5. Food Allergies; people with certain food allergies are advised to avoid foods containing eggs, gluten, fish, soy, wheat, dairy, nuts etc, then make up for this nutritional loss by taking supplements as recommended by a certified dietician.

6. The diet is difficult to modify; the low-FODMAP diet does not give room for a middle ground, it's either all or nothing because you have to go through the elimination phase first before trying to reintroduce some foods back into your diet, there is no room for compromise in that and it can be even more Challenging for people with additional nutritional restrictions, but it isn't impossible.

Chapter Five: Recommended Foods For The Low Fodmap Diet

The biggest dilemma people with IBS face is what to eat. Think about it. When you have a nightmare where you found yourself in a really dark place, for a couple of days, even months, you'll find that you get uncomfortable in dark environments. But what do you do? Will always walk around with a torch? Or do you face your fears? It's the same in this case, we all need food to survive, so you can't totally avoid food for fear of triggering your symptoms. But there's a solution, and I am sure you will be glad to hear it. Along with the elimination and reintroduction phase, it is also very helpful to know the foods recommended for the low-FODMAP diet, because it is sometimes hard to gain relief from IBS symptoms but very easy to trigger them. So what are they? What are these heaven sent foods that can give you relief at last?

Surprisingly, they are not as few as you might have been led to believe, if you follow the diet right, you might not even miss those foods that wreak havoc on your bowels. Should you even?

Low-FODMAP foods;

- Low-FODMAP fruits
- Most seeds and nuts
- Low-FODMAP veggies
- Most non-dairy milk
- Low-FODMAP grains
- Some sweeteners
- Tofu and tempeh
- Fish, meat and eggs
- Lactose-free dairy products
- Low-FODMAP certified foods

There are a lot of low-FODMAP vegetables some of which are; cabbage, potatoes, bok choy, sweet potatoes, carrots, kale, turnips, collard greens, bell peppers, lettuce, squash, eggplant and arugula.

Low-FODMAP Fruits

I know what you are thinking, how in the clouds do you tell a low-FODMAP fruit from a high-FODMAP fruit? Well, you don't have to go to the lab to get it tested, that's for sure. All you need to know is that low-FODMAP fruits are low in fructans and fructose. With this little information and some research, I am sure you'll learn thats fruits like; oranges, honeydew melons, kiwis, bananas, cantaloupe, lemons, blueberries, pineapples, grapes, strawberries and raspberries are all low-FODMAP and completely acceptable on a low-FODMAP diet.

Most Seeds And Nuts

We all know the nutritional values of nuts and seeds and thankfully, most of them are low-FODMAP. Afew of which are; Pecans, chia seeds, macadamia nuts, brazil nuts, pumpkin seeds, pine nuts, sunflower seeds, walnuts, sesame seeds, and peanuts.\

Low-FODMAP Veggies

It may seem a bit overwhelming with the wide variety of vegetables we have, but examples of a few very common low-FODMAP vegetables are; carrots, cabbage, broccoli, eggplant, kale, ginger, okra, radish, seaweed, yam, tomatoes, english and baby spinach, potatoes, cucumbers and fennels.

Most Non-Dairy Milk

Since most dairy milk are notorious for triggering IBS symptoms, here are a few alternatives; coconut milk (in very small amounts, hemp milk, almond milk, and rice milk.

Low-FODMAP Grains

While there are a couple grains that are not accepted on a low-FODMAP diet, others like; quinoa, amaranth, bulgar (in small amounts), oats, brown rice, and spelt are safe because most of them are gluten free.

Some Sweeteners

A lot of sweeteners these days are either high in fructose or fructans or both, and as you know, those are enemies to the low-FODMAP diet. So, what do my fellow compadres with sweet teeth do? Live a life with no sweetness? Waste away and sink deeper into bitter misery? No! We want low-FODMAP sweeteners! We have our pitchforks and torches at the ready, we will do what we must! Fortunately, we won't have to resort to violence, low-FODMAP sweeteners like white sugar, powdered sugar, maple syrup, brown sugar and a couple of artificial sweeteners have jumped in and saved the day.

Tofu And Tempeh

These can serve as great sources of protein for people on the low-FODMAP diet. Vegans can also use them as an alternative for high-FODMAP legumes to make up for their protein requirements.

Fish, Meat And Eggs

Good news! O ye meat and fish lovers! All other non-dairy animal products are acceptable on a low-FODMAP diet. So you can join in and devour that roasted turkey during Thanksgiving, some chicken wings with friends, barbecued beef with the besties, pork rind on a nice weekend and eggs for breakfast! Hurray! Although, you are advised to avoid processed meats like corned beef and sausages. I am sure you can live with that.

Lactose-Free Dairy Products

The main reason why dairy products are considered high-FODMAP is because they contain lactose. So if you are in the mood for some yoghurt or ice cream , or you have a bowl of cereal heaped with milk in front of you, you might want to think again. You don't necessarily have to do without, you can opt for lactose-free options. You can also have some cheeses like parmesan and mozzarella on the diet.

Low-FODMAP Certified Foods

A few companies (e.g kelloggs) produce low-FODMAP certified foods like bars, cereals , snacks, bread and more. You can get them in many grocery stores.

With the recommended foods above, your Low-FODMAP diet should move comfortably. Although do not exceed the recommended amounts of these foods because a couple of Low-FODMAP foods put together can quickly become a high-FODMAP meal.

How To Make Life Easier On The Diet?

No diet is easy because you are being drawn out of your comfort zone. Although, it is for the greater good. Even though the low-FODMAP diet can be a bit challenging, here are a few tips to make the diet easy peesy;

1. Variety is the spice of life; explore new types of food in this diet. Do not just stick to those that you are familiar with. If you eat the same thing over and over again, it will soon get boring and thereby making the diet more difficult to stick to. Challenge yourself to eat a little of everything so that you can make up your daily nutritional needs.
2. Do not eat too many fruits at a go; I am sure you need no explanation on this one, because too many fruits are high in fructose or fructans or both, so? In this case, less is more.
3. Do not drink too much alcohol; While it might be fun to club and party to your heart's content, the aftermath is not always pleasant for your bowels. So, have some pity, if not for yourself, but for your poor, abused bowels.
4. Stay hydrated; Make water your best friend. It helps move stool easier in your bowels. So, Drop that soda and take a sip

of water. Who knows? You might just be one sip away from sweet relief

5. Try to space out your meals; A couple of hours between meals is sure to ease your abdominal pain , so wait at least 3-4 hours after each meal or if you can wait, you can make it longer.

6. Buy seasonal produce; it is highly recommended that you consume only fresh fruits and vegetables, but they tend to be very expensive. So, to minimize cost, you could try buying those that are in season, they are usually cheaper.

7. Buy only Low-FODMAP certified foods; sometimes you crave the things you used to have, don't worry, it's perfectly normal. When you need pasta, cereals, grains and breads, opt for those that have been certified by the Monash University.

Dietary Modifications

A lot of people with IBD or IBS have one allergy or the other or food intolerance. Some of the most allergens are; shellfish, gluten, dairy, nuts and soy. So, below are a few tips on how to modify the low-FODMAP diet to suit your allergy.

1. Gluten-free; Although the low-FODMAP diet may contain gluten, you can totally omit those foods from your diet without any harm. So, instead of rye or barley, you can use quinoa or brown rice instead.

2. Vegan; Vegans normally rely on foods like split peas, beans and lentils as a source of protein, but these foods are high-FODMAP, which makes it very difficult for vegans to get enough protein on a low-FODMAP diet. To make up for that, foods like quinoa, tempeh, tofu, seeds and nuts are recommended.

3. Children; Children have a lot of nutritional needs, that is why many diets aren't recommended for children, and the low-FODMAP diet isn't an exception. Research hasn't yet been made in regards to the safety of a low-FODMAP diet for children, so if your child has IBS related symptoms, you

might want to talk to a pediatrician. If a supervised Low-FODMAP diet is suggested, then you might want to try it, only until your child feels better.

4. Soy-free; foods containing soy are not allowed on a low-FODMAP diet, so if you use soy as a source of protein, you might want to try something else.Animal products or nuts are also good options.

5. Pregnancy; No research has been done as of yet as regards to a low-FODMAP diet in pregnancy, so it is not recommended. Although if you have any IBS related symptoms in pregnancy, you might want to avoid or reduce your intake of the foods that you are sensitive to.

6. Dairy-free; The low-FODMAP diet is mostly dairy free, but to make it completely so, you should skip the lactose-free products and soft-cheeses and opt for Low-FODMAP non-dairy milk instead.

7. Vegetarians; Vegetarians can consume foods containing dairy products, unlike their vegan counterparts, but since there are restrictions on dairy products for the low-FODMAP diet, vegetarians are advised to go for lactose-free dairy or non-dairy products and also consume enough low-FODMAP proteins.

8. Allergen-Friendly; Adopting an allergen-friendly low-FODMAP diet can be really challenging, but not impossible. If you are allergic to some foods such as shellfish or tree nuts, just avoid them, they won't affect how you react to other foods.

Chapter Six: Recommended Supplements

People on the low-fodmap diet have nutritional needs that need to be met, this is due to the restrictive nature of the diet, and the logical solution as you well know would be supplements, but the question is, what type of supplements?

Fiber

Fibre is one of the important components of plant based foods (e.g vegetables, legumes, fruits and grains) that are indigestible, but it performs a lot of other functions in the body that are beneficial to gut health. There are different types of fibre, and they are; prebiotics, soluble and insoluble fibre, but what I am sure you'd like to know is if fiber supplements can help people with ibs who are on a low or modified FODMAP diet. Well, we'll get to that in about a minute, let's find out more about fibres first.

Where is fibre found?

A lot of foods naturally contain a mixture of many different fibres, so getting fibre from food sources like vegetables, fruits, legumes, wholegrains and nuts is relatively easy. Fibre supplements on the other hand contain one particular type of fibre and may be used when a person can't get enough fibre through food alone.

Advantages

Fibre plays a huge role in our bodies, including everything from normalising cholesterol and blood sugar levels, providing fuel for the gut microbiome, controlling bowel habits, etc. each fibre has its function, one might have amazing blood sugar regulating properties and have zero effect where the bowels are concerned, while the other might flourish in that department.

The Risk Of A Diet Low In Fibre

When you eliminate foods from your diet, you put yourself at risk of reducing important micro or macronutrients , amongst which we have fibre. When you go on a low-fodmap diet, there is a risk that you would reduce your fibre intake, this happens mostly because the key sources of fibre like barley, wheat, legumes and rhy are limited. The possibility of fiber supplements working for people with IBS depends on the function of the fibre contained in the supplements and its physiological characteristics. For example,its solubility in water i.e its fermentability and water holding abilities or the possibility of it producing gas in the large intestine. There have been several researches carried out concerning the effects of fibre supplements on people with IBS, but as of yet, none have been conclusive. So, I am going to share a few fibre supplements and observations shared by a couple of people who used them. So with that and the help of your dietician, you'll be able to figure which would work best for you.

Type Of Fibre Supplement	Observation
Wheat Dextrin	There has been no research in relation to IBS.
Wheat Bran	It is unable to normalize bowel movements and as such may worsen symptoms of IBS.
Sterculia	It is non-fermentable and has shown to be beneficial to people with IBS because it helps with stool softening. Although, further studies need to be carried out on

	this.
Partially Hydrolysed Guar Gum (PHGG)	It has prebiotic properties which promote gut health, and has shown to help relieve IBS related diarrhoea and constipation although the research isn't conclusive.
Inulin	It is highly fermentable which may cause IBS symptoms to worsen.
Linseeds	Although research is not conclusive, it has been observed that at least two tablespoons may relieve IBS related constipation, bloating and abdominal pain.
Psyllium	Although psyllium may not be tolerated by a lot of people, research shows that it may help relieve IBS related constipation
Resistant Starch	It ferments slowly along the length of the large intestine, so it might not cause as much discomfort as the highly fermentable ones.
Oats	May help improve bloating, constipation and abdominal pain in people with IBS, but studies are not yet

	conclusive.
Fructooligosaccharides (FOS)/galactooligosaccharides (GOS)	These are highly fermentable and may worsen IBS symptoms.
methylcellulose	It does not ferment and as such may help relieve IBS symptoms.

Digestive Enzymes

What are digestive enzymes? They are those little worker bees that help us digest our food. So,what happens to people who do not produce enough of them? Ofcourse, they may have a hard time digesting certain foods and as a result may have very painful symptoms due to food that travels undigested to the large intestine. It is in cases like these that diarrhoea, bloating and gas tend to arise. Most times people with IBS lack the digestive enzymes required to digest certain foods, that is why they react so badly to them and as such, digestive enzymes might be recommended as a form of treatment through supplementation. Here are a list of available digestive enzymes and their possible uses;

Enzymes	Possible Uses
Xylose Isomerase	This is one of the enzymes that are not produced by the body. Its function is to convert fructose to glucose, which would help ease digestive problems and aid in the absorption of

	disaccharides.
Lactase (B-galactosidase)	This enzyme is in charge of breaking down lactose into its smaller components(e.g galactose) which in turn helps improve digestion.
Pancrelipase	This enzyme helps to break down fats into more soluble components. Although, fat is not a fodmap, but a lot of IBS sufferers have a hard time digesting high fat meals
Alpha-galactosidase	This enzyme helps break down certain oligosaccharides such as stachyose and raffinose or (GOS) galacto-oligosaccharides which is found in some whole grains, beans, cabbage, broccoli, peas and some other vegetables. It is not produced in the body, that is why GOS can travel to the large intestine without being digested.

Probiotics

There has been a lot of talk about the benefits of probiotics and its effects on gut health, but is it safe to take them when on the low-FODMAP diet? But how do you know which one to take and when? Let's get these questions answered.

What Are Probiotics?

Probiotics are defined as live microorganisms that have health benefits when given to the host in adequate amounts. Some would refer to probiotics as "good bacteria" in contrasts to its pathogenic counterparts. You should note the word "live" in the definition, this means that the bacteria is administered alive because it needs to survive the journey through the GIT into your colon.

Since the pH of the stomach is very high (i.e acidic), not all bacteria can survive the tedious and acidic journey long enough to be of any benefit to you. Although, quantity also matters as just a few won't really do anything.

How do they work?

Probiotics interact with the gut in several ways, being administered a particular type of probiotic might promote the growth of a type of good-bacteria that you may be lacking. It is common knowledge that people on a low-FODMAP diet tend to have reduced numbers of bifidobacteria due to a reduction in prebiotic fiber, so a probiotic supplement containing this species of bacteria may help maintain gut health.

Certain strains of bacteria may also promote production of B-galactosidase which may aid in the absorption of lactose in some individuals, while others might impede the growth of bacteria causing inflammation in the gut.

In addition, probiotics can increase production of short-chain fatty acids in the colon, which can decrease intestinal pH and enhance the barrier function of the epithelium (these are the cells that line the stomach and intestines)[3].

These effects of probiotics on the gut may result in a marked improvement in people with IBS symptoms such as improved stool consistency, reduced gas and bloating, improved diarrhoea or constipation, decreased abdominal pain and an improved quality of life.

It may be possible for probiotics to prove more effective in people who have microbille alterations like in the case of people with

Post-infectious IBS.

Which Probiotic To Take?

IBS symptoms are diverse and affect each person differently, and as such, what may work for one might have no effect in another. Although more research is being done on gut health in relation to probiotics, we still haven't discovered as much as we would like to. So, we still do not know a lot of things.

How effective the probiotics prove would be determined by your diet, your unique gut microbiota, genetics, levels of exercise, type of IBS related symptoms you have and age.

When purchasing a probiotic supplement, you should consider the following;

- Dose; all probiotic supplements have the number of colony forming units (CFUs) written on them. CFUs are the number of bacteria that can live and reproduce to form a new colony or group of identical bacteria. Like i mentioned before, numbers matter. Without numbers, it would be like going to fight an army by yourself with weapons or armor.
- Brands; some brands include prebiotics in their supplements which may contain some fiber like GOS or inulin which have high FODMAP content, so be sure to carefully read the labels.
- Where to buy;thankfully, you can find probiotics in many pharmacies or chemist and also in some natural food stores.

When To Consider Taking Probiotic supplements?

The Monash University recommends that you wait after the first two phases of the low-FODMAp diet before taking any probiotic supplement, as you might be unable to tell if they are helping or triggering your symptoms. Introducing probiotics during the elimination phase is a very bad idea as it may worsen your symptoms and result an issue you didn't have before.

If a dietician or doctor prescribes probiotics for you during the elimination phase, you might want to discuss the pros and cons before doing so or better still, find a better solution.

How To Take Probiotics

Although probiotics are safe enough to be taken daily, it is important that you read the product labels or any additional information that comes with the supplement before taking it and also use them as prescribed by your healthcare provider. Just bear in mind that sometimes, more isn't better. In your zeal to get better, you might end up doing more harm than good.

Note that it is recommended that you don't take probiotic supplements on an empty stomach as food may help serve as a buffer against the acidity of the stomach, which would give the bacteria a fighting chance to make it through the GIT. Also, if you are expecting immediate results after taking probiotic supplements, you will be disappointed as it takes a minimum of four weeks for results to show.

NOTE: Probiotic supplements are not recommended in adults with immuno-compromised health related issues and in children as there might be adverse side effects.

Chapter Seven: Low-Fodmap Breakfast Recipes

Hey! Yes you! I have something amazing to share with you and i promise it is going to be better than the last episode of your favorite telenovela. You can now eat your favorite breakfast without worrying about your IBS. No kidding! With the low-FODMAP breakfast recipes shared below, you'll feel as good as new. Aren't you excited? So, let's make some breakfast!

Low-Fodmap Frittata

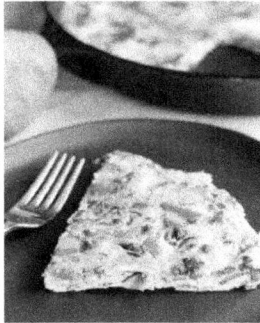

- Prep Time: 5 Minutes
- Cook Time: 20 Minutes
- Yield: 8 Servings
- Calories: 169 Calories
- Nutrition Fact: **Sugars;** 2g **Proteins;** 8g **Fats;** 11g **Carbs; 7g**

What you'll Need

- Some oil for frying
- Six(6) cherry tomatoes
- Two(2) slices of ham
- Eight(8) medium sized eggs

- Two(2) handfuls of spinach

Instructions

1. Put the spinach into a small pan, add about three tablespoons of water, set over medium heat and allow to simmer for 2-3 minutes or until completely wilted.
2. Crack the eggs into a medium sized mixing bowl and beat it lightly with a fork or whisk.
3. Cut the ham into little bits, then pour it into the egg mix.
4. Put in the wilted spinach and stir until fully combined.
5. Season with pepper and salt to taste.
6. Pour some oil into a medium sized frying pan, set on medium heat and allow to simmer for 5 minutes.
7. Pour in the egg mixture and make sure it is spread out evenly, then allow to cook for 5 minutes on each side.
8. Do not flip the frittata even when it starts to look cook around the edges, check the top to see if it is cooked, if it is not, then leave it for a few more minutes.
9. Turn off heat, then use a spatula put the frittata on a flat plate.
10. Use a sharp knife to cut the frittata into slices.
11. Serve hot or cold. Enjoy!

NOTE: You can serve your frittatas with a little something on the side if you plan to eat them immediately, if not, allow them to cool for a bit, then put each slice into small tupperware boxes and put them in the fridge until you are ready.

Low-Fodmap Banana Pancakes

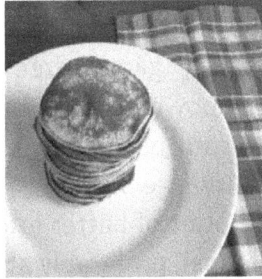

- Prep Time: 5 Minutes
- Cook Time: 20 Minutes
- Yield: 2 Servings
- Calories: 278 Calories
- Nutrition Fact:**Sugars;** 2g **Proteins;** 14g **Fats;** 12g **Carbs;** 30g

What You'll Need

- Two(2) large eggs
- One(1) tablespoon of brown sugar
- A quarter teaspoon of ground nutmeg
- 160 grams of banana (firm with no brown spots)
- Half a teaspoon of ground cinnamon
- Two(2) tablespoons of gluten free all purpose flour
- A pinch
- Three(3) tablespoons of dairy-free spread (butter or olive oil for cooking)
- A quarter teaspoon of baking powder
- Two(2) large eggs

Toppings

- Six(6) tablespoons of lactose free yogurt or coconut yoghurt
- A pinch of confectioners sugar
- Ten blueberries

Instructions

1. Peel the bananas and put them into a large bowl, then mash them or process them using an immersion blender until smooth.
2. Crack in the eggs and mix to combine.
3. Add the salt, nutmeg, gluten free flour, brown sugar, cinnamon and baking powder, stir until well combined.
4. Put a large cast iron pan over medium heat, add a tablespoon of the dairy-free butter.
5. Pour a measured amount of batter into the pan (to get your desired size of pancakes), preferably about 3-4 tablespoons.
6. Allow the batter to cook over medium heat for 3-5 minutes or until tiny bubbles start to form on the top.
7. Raise the sides of the pancake a bit to check if the underside golden brown, if it is, flip it.
8. Cook on both sides until they are well cooked and lightly browned.
9. Serve with blueberries or low-FODMAP yoghurt and enjoy!

NOTE: If at any point the pancakes start to stick to the pan, you can add a dash of dairy-free spread to grease the pan a bit, and if the pancakes appear to burn too quickly, reduce the heat and leave the pan for a bit before pouring in more batter.

Low-Fodmap Quinoa Porridge

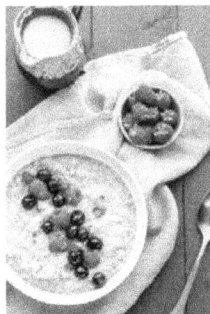

- Prep Time: 2 Mins
- Cook Time: 25 Minutes
- Yield: 2 Servings
- Calories: 281 Calories
- Nutrition Fact: **Sugars;** 15.7g **Proteins;** 6.7g **Fats;** 6.2g **Carbs;** 50.2g

What You'll Need

- Twenty(20) blueberries (fresh or frozen)
- A quarter teaspoon of ground cinnamon
- one(1) teaspoon of neutral oil (sunflower, rice bran, canola)
- Ten(10) raspberries
- Four(4) teaspoons of pure maple syrup
- Half a cup of quinoa
- A cup of water
- A cup of low-FODMAP milk

Instructions

1. Pour the quinoa into a fine mesh sieve and rinse under cold running water for a minute or two.
2. Put the rinsed quinoa into a medium sized saucepan and add a spoonful or two of neutral oil.

3. Set the saucepan over low heat and allow the quinoa to cook until it completely loses all moisture and starts to toast (i.e about 2 minutes), then add water.
4. Bring the mixture to a rolling boil, then turn down the heat, then cook covered for another 10-15 minutes until fluffy and soft.
5. Stir, then drain of excess water if need be.
6. Add cinnamon, low-FODMAP milk and maple syrup, stir to combine.
7. Add a bit more milk if the previously added one dries up fast, stir and allow to simmer for a little over 5 minutes.
8. Serve the porridge into bowls and serve topped with blueberries and raspberries

NOTE: You can also store the porridge in a glass lidded jar for up to a week. All you need to do is keep the ingredients in step 6 above until you are ready to eat.

Low-Fodmap Tortilla

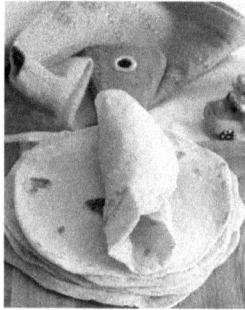

- Prep Time: 5 Minutes
- Cook Time: 5 Minutes
- Yield: 1 Serving
- Calories: 177 Calories
- Nutrition Fact: **Sugars;** 3g **Proteins;** 1.8g **Fats;** 2g **Carbs;** 35g

What You'll Need

- A quarter cup of water
- A cup of gluten free all purpose flour
- Half a tablespoon of extra virgin olive oil
- A pinch of salt

Instructions

1. Put oil, flour, water and salt into a food processor and process until a thick smooth dough is formed, or pour all the ingredients into a large mixing bowl and knead by hand.
2. Cut the dough in two and place a piece between two pieces of parchment paper, roll out the dough until it is well thinned out.
3. Gently peel off the pieces of parchment, then repeat the process for the rest of the dough.
4. Place a non-stick pan on low heat and gently place the thinned out dough in it, then allow to cook for 1-2 minutes or until the underside is lightly browned, then flip it and cook the top(now facing down) for another 1-2 minutes.
5. Serve and enjoy!

NOTE: You can alternatively leave the piece of parchment at the top of the thinned out dough until the bottom part is thoroughly cooked before peeling off the piece of parchment at the top, then flip and allow to cook until lightly browned. Although you may have to be very watchful as the parchment paper is flammable, so try not to let it come in direct contact with the flame. This method also helps the dough not swell too much, which makes the tortillas very flat and pliable. Also note that the tortillas will harden if they are overcooked, so set a timer if you are not sure if you will be able to keep to time.

Low-Fodmap Pumpkin Pancake

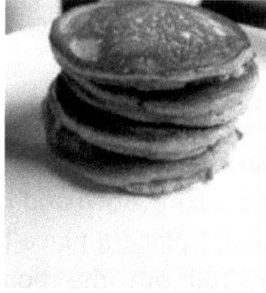

- Prep Time: 20 Minutes
- Cook Time: 30 Minutes
- Yield: 6 Servings
- Calories: 531 Calories
- Nutrition Fact: **Sugars**;21.2g **Proteins**;11g **Fats**;24.3g **Carbs**;65.1g

What You'll Need

- Half a teaspoon of ground nutmeg
- Four(4) tablespoons of water
- A cup of fresh pumpkin puree or canned pumpkin
- Two(2) teaspoons of baking powder
- Half a teaspoon of ground ginger
- Two(2) medium sized eggs
- Three(3) tablespoons of brown sugar
- A quarter teaspoon of salt
- Two(2) teaspoons of ground cinnamon
- One(1) teaspoon of baking soda
- Two(2) tablespoons of neutral oil
- Two(2) cups of low-FODMAP milk
- Two(2) cups of gluten free all purpose flour

To Serve;

44

- Four(4) tablespoons of pure maple syrup (optional)
- Two(2) tablespoons of pumpkin seeds(optional)

Instructions

1. Preheat your oven to 120F.
2. To make the pumpkin puree(i.e if you do not already have some made); wash, peel and deseed a medium sized pumpkin, cut it into small bite sized pieces, then put it into a medium sized steel bowl with about 4 or 5 tablespoons of water, then put it into the oven and allow it to wilt for 5-10 minutes or until the pumpkin appears very soft.
3. Rinse the pumpkins in cold water for a while, drain it and set it aside to cool for a couple of minutes.
4. Once cool, transfer into a blender jar, add about three or four tablespoons of water and process until smooth, if the puree appears too thick, add a tablespoon of water and puree again. Repeat this process until you have the right consistency (i.e not too thick or too runny).
5. Put the brown sugar, baking soda, salt, gluten free flour, cinnamon, baking powder, ginger and nutmeg into a large mixing bowl, stir until well combined.
6. Put the egg, low-FODMAP milk and neutral oil into another bowl and stir until well combined.
7. Pour the pureed pumpkin into the wet ingredients and stir until well mixed.
8. Pour the wet ingredients into the dry ingredients and stir to combine, if the mixture appears too thick, add a few dollops of low-FODMAP milk.
9. Put about a tablespoon of neutral oil into a large non-stick pan and set on medium heat, allow the oil to simmer for a minute, then pour a quarter cup of batter into the pan.
10. Cook for three minutes on each side or use a spatula to slightly lift the side of the pancakes, peak under to check if it is golden brown, if it is, flip it and allow the other side cook until it is golden brown.

11. Place the cooked pancakes unto a baking sheet or steel plate and put into the oven to keep it warm while you cook the rest of the batter.
12. Serve hot with a banana, bacon, maple syrup, or toasted pumpkin seeds.

NOTE: Be mindful of how much extra milk you add to your mixture if not you might soon find that the batter is a bit too runny. If this happens, add a tablespoon of gluten free flour, stir then repeat until you have your desired consistency. Enjoy!

Low-Fodmap Pikelets

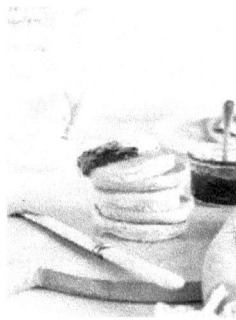

- Prep Time: 10 Minutes
- Cook Time: 15 Minutes
- Yield: 16 Servings
- Calories: 116 Calories
- Nutrition Fact: **Sugars**;9.4g **Proteins**;1.4g **Fats**;3.8g **Carbs**;18.7g

What You'll Need

- A cup of low-FODMAP milk
- 175 grams of gluten free all-purpose flour
- Two(2) teaspoons of dairy free spread
- One (1) medium sized egg

- Two(2) tablespoons of white sugar
- One(1) teaspoon of pure vanilla extract
- Three(3) teaspoons of baking powder

For serving;

- Eight(8) tablespoons of strawberry jam
- Half a cup of regular fat whipped cream

Instructions

1. Put the white sugar, baking powder and gluten free flour into a medium sized mixing bowl, stir until well combined, then make a well in the center, by turning your hand continuously in the middle of the bowl until a groove is formed or you could just use your hands or a spoon to spread out the flour mix.
2. Add the egg, milk and vanilla, whisk the ingredients together until an almost lump free batter is formed.
3. To check that the batter is the right consistency, dip the whisk into the mixture, then raise it high, almost to your eye level, the dough shouldn't fall right off the whisk, it should trickle off slowly and leave a little swirl or tail at the top of the batter. If it doesn't do this, all you have to do is add a few spoonfuls of low-FODMAP milk, but it all depends on the amount of gluten flour used.
4. Put a small amount of dairy-free spread into a small non-stick pan and set over medium heat, allow to simmer for a few seconds then add about three tablespoons of batter into the pan.
5. Cook for 3-5 minutes or small bubbles start to form at the top, flip and also cook the same amount of time or until both sides are golden.
6. Put the pikelet onto a plate and repeat the process for the rest of the batter.
7. Serve warm with a generous amount of whipped cream and strawberry jam.
8. Enjoy!

NOTE: If you find that you have an excess amount of oil or melted dairy-free spread in your pan, tilt the pan over a steel bowl (if it's too hot, it might burn a plastic plate), let the excess trickle into the steel bowl, then set the pan back on the heat. This is done to prevent your pikelets from cooking unevenly or burning.

Low-Fodmap Omelet

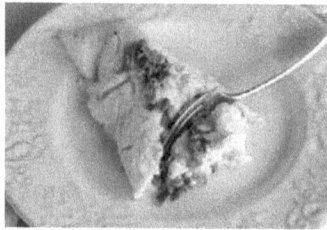

- Prep Time: 5 Minutes
- Cook Time: 10 Minutes
- Yield: 1 Serving
- Calories: 397 Calories
- Nutrition Fact: **Sugars**;1g **Proteins**;16g **Fats**;33g **Carbs**;5g

What You'll Need

- A cup of oyster mushrooms (cleaned and chopped)
- Three(3) medium sized eggs
- Two(2) tablespoons of dairy-free spread
- A pinch of kosher salt
- One(1) teaspoon of water
- A small pinch of freshly ground black pepper

Instructions

1. Put about a tablespoon of dairy-free spread into a non-stick pan and allow to simmer for a few seconds until bubbly.
2. Throw in the mushrooms and saute for 2-3 minutes until the mushrooms start to soften.

3. Add pepper and salt (and more if you feel the need), stir then scrape the mushroom into a small bowl.
4. So as not to give yourself too many things to wash, wipe out the skillet and add the rest of the dairy-free spread into it.
5. Set over medium heat and allow to melt.
6. Crack the egg into a bowl and beat them slightly, then pour them into the heated pan.
7. Use your spatula or spoon to carefully draw in the edges of the egg so that the uncooked parts can flow towards the edge of the pan, if you find that to be a bit difficult, told the pan side ways to force the uncooked part of the egg to go to the edges of the pan.
8. Pour Half of the cooked mushrooms for into the egg mixture, then keep the rest to top the eggs after they are cooked.
9. Cook for 2-3 minutes on each side or until the egg is a little moist, but not watery or runny and not too dry too.
10. Fold in both sides of the egg and use a spatula to transfer it into a plate.
11. Top with the rest of the mushrooms and serve hot.

NOTE: You can also use the tips in this recipe to make any other omelet recipe you might have in mind. You can switch the mushrooms for a bit of green or red bell peppers, feta or cooked spinach. How about a bit of dried herbs or spices in the eggs? The possibilities are endless! Just make sure whatever alternatives you use a low-FODMAP.

Low-Fodmap Breakfast Squares

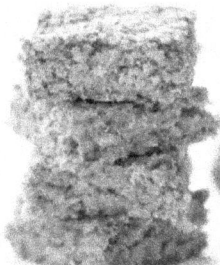

- Prep Time: 10 Minutes
- Cook Time: 30 Minutes
- Yield: 16 Servings
- Calories: 264 Calories
- Nutrition Fact:**Sugars; 7.8g Proteins; 13g Fats; 8g Carbs; 28g**

What You'll Need

- Half a cup of sugar
- One(1) teaspoon of baking powder
- One(1) cup of gluten free oats
- Half a teaspoon of salt
- One(1) cup of cooked quinoa
- Two (2) ripe bananas (mashed)
- A quarter cup of peanut butter
- One(1) teaspoon of pure vanilla extract
- A quarter cup of raisins or chocolate chips (optional)
- Two(2) eggs
- Two(2) teaspoons of cinnamon

Instructions

1. Preheat your oven to 350F.
2. Grease a baking pan with cooking spray or line it with pieces of parchment paper.
3. Put all the ingredients into a large mixing bowl and mix using a whisk until well combined, or you might as well put ok the ingredients into a food processor and blend until well combined.
4. Pour batter into greased pan and use the flat side of a spoon to level the top until smooth.
5. Bake for 25-30 minutes or until firm and well browned on the top. You can also check with a fork or toothpick to be sure, if it comes out clean, then your treat is ready.
6. Remove from the oven and set aside to cool, still in the pan.
7. Remove from the pan and set atop a flat plate and cut them into squares.

8. Put into an airtight jar or container, then refrigerate and enjoy at your leisure!

NOTES: To cook the quinoa, put twice the amount of water into a pot of water, set over medium heat and bring to a boil. Rinse the quinoa under cold running water, then add it to the pot of boiling water. Cook covered for 10 minutes, then reduce the heat and allow to simmer for 5 minutes until it loses all moisture. Make sure to stir occasionally so that the quinoa doesn't stick to the bottom of the pot.

Low-Fodmap Breakfast Bites

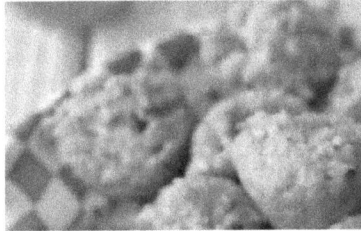

- Prep Time: 15 Minutes
- Cook Time: 55 Minutes
- Yield: 10 Servings
- Calories: 212 Calories
- Nutrition Fact:**Sugars;** 6.3g **Proteins;** 16g **Fats;** 5g **Carbs;** 16.4g

What You'll Need

- Three(3) medium sized eggs
- One(1) cup quinoa (uncooked)
- Pepper and salt to taste
- Two(2) cups of vegetable broth
- Half a teaspoon of dried oregano
- One(1) cup of bagged, cut leaf spinach
- A quarter cup of chopped scallions (green part only)

- One(1) cup of crumbled feta cheese

Instructions

1. Preheat your oven to 350F.
2. Grease a couple of mini muffin pans with cooking spray or line them with small pieces of parchment paper.
3. To cook the quinoa; Rinse the quinoa under cold running water, drain it and put it into a pot.
4. Pour in the vegetable broth and set the pot over medium heat and bring to a boil.
5. Once boiled, reduce the heat, stir then cover and allow to simmer for 15 minutes or until it loses all moisture, then remove from heat.
6. Put all the ingredients into a large mixing bowl and stir until well combined using a wooden spoon.
7. Scoop the mixture into the muffin pans using an ice cream scoop or a tablespoon.
8. Bake for 25-30 minutes or until well browned and firm on the top.
9. Remove from the oven and set on cooling racks, still in the muffin pans to cool for 5-10 minutes.
10. Gentle pry out the bites from the muffin tins using a butter knife.
11. Serve and enjoy immediately, or put them into air tight jars or containers and refrigerate.
12. Enjoy!

Low-Fodmap Egg Cups

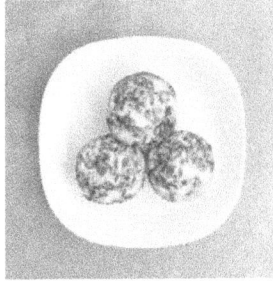

- Prep Time: 10 Minutes
- Cook Time: 30 Minutes
- Yield: 3 Servings
- Calories: 338 Calories
- Nutrition Fact:**Sugars;** 5g **Proteins;** 19.8g **Fats;** 6.2g **Carbs;** 5g

What You'll Need

- Half a cup of spinach leaves (stems removed and chopped)
- One(3) medium sized egg
- Half a tablespoon of crumbled feta cheese
- One(1) cherry tomato
- One(1) tablespoon of lactose-free milk

Instructions

1. Preheat your oven to 325F.
2. Grease 3 muffin pans with cooking spray or line them with small pieces of parchment paper.
3. Crack an egg into each of the muffin pan, pour un a tablespoon of lactose free milk and stir gently with a teaspoon.
4. Add the rest of the ingredients, using a spoon to press them down to give enough room for the rest of the ingredients before proceeding to the next.

5. Bake for 10-30 minutes until the egg cups are firm and golden.

Chapter Eight: Low-Fodmap Lunch Recipes

Yum! Yum! Time for some tasty lunch. Why aren't you happy? Everyone with IBS loves a good Low-FODMAP lunch. Oh? No cooking skills? Worry not, because Aron saves the day yet again! These recipes are totally beginner friendly and are sure to make you feel better in no time!

Low-Fodmap Macaroni

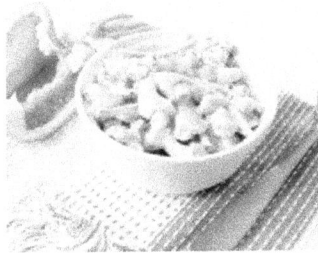

- Prep Time: 10 Minutes
- Cook Time: 10 Servings
- Yield: 10 Servings
- Calories: 152 Calories
- Nutrition Fact: **Sugar**; 2g **Proteins**;7g **Fats**;4g **Carbs**;21g

Ingredients

- One (1) tablespoon of mustard
- Half a cup of non-dairy yoghurt
- A quarter cup of chopped fresh chives
- A quarter cup of mayonnaise
- A cup of gluten free macaroni or lentil macaroni
- One(1) teaspoon of kosher salt
- Two(2) tablespoons of Apple cider vinegar

- Half a cup of shredded carrots
- A quarter teaspoon of black pepper
- One(1) cup of chopped green pepper

Instructions

1. Put the vinegar, yoghurt, salt and pepper, mayonnaise and mustard into a large bowl, stir until well combined, then add green pepper, chives, carrots and macaroni, stir to combine using a wooden spoon.
2. Serve immediately or put into a plastic container and store in the fridge until you are ready.

Low-Fodmap Quinoa Salad

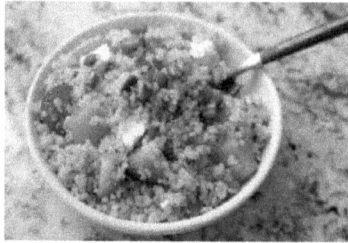

- Prep Time: 10 Minutes
- Cook Time: 20 Minutes
- Yield: 6 Servings
- Calories: 229 Calories
- Nutrition Fact:**Sugars;** 4g **Proteins;** 12g **Fats;** 6g **Carbs;** 31g

Ingredients

- One(1) cup of feta cheese
- One(1) cup of uncooked quinoa
- A quarter teaspoon of black pepper
- Two(2) cups of vegetable broth
- Three(3) tablespoons of lemon juice
- One(1) cup of chopped tomatoes
- One(1) teaspoon of dried basil

- One(1) cup of chopped cucumbers
- A quarter teaspoon of salt
- One(1) teaspoon of dried oregano
- Two(2) tablespoons of extra virgin olive oil
- One(1) cup of chopped bell peppers
- Half a cup of diced spring onions (green part only)

Instructions

1. Pour the vegetable broth into a medium sized saucepan and set over medium heat, bring to a boil, add the quinoa then reduce the heat and allow to simmer for 15 minutes until the broth is completely absorbed.
2. Put the quinoa into a large bowl and set aside to cool until ready for use.
3. Wash all the vegetables, then cut them into small squares or bite sized pieces, also cut the feta cheese into small pieces.
4. Once the vegetables are ready, throw them into the bowl quinoa along with the rest of the ingredients. Mix until well incorporated.
5. Taste and make any necessary adjustments in the seasoning.

NOTES: You can use garlic infused oil if you do not have olive oil, it has a unique taste that will give this recipe a wonderful flavour, you can also use both by using one tablespoons of each. The oil has a very concentrated taste and smell so you might try a tablespoon or two, then add as you go if you feel the need. You should also note that the white parts of the spring onions contain fructans that is why I recommended the green parts for this recipe., So it might be helpful to you if you are sensitive to fructans or if you are in you are in your elimination phase and are still not sure of what triggers your symptoms.

Low-Fodmap Curly Fries

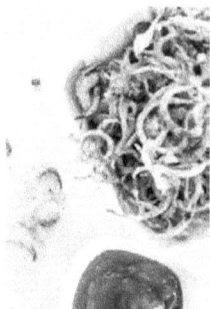

- Prep Time: 20 Minutes
- Cook Time: 25 Minutes
- Yield: 4 Servings
- Calories: 185 Calories
- Nutrition Fact: **Sugars**; 1.8g **Proteins**;4.4g **Fats**; 2.7g **Carbs**; 36.9g

What You'll Need

- A pinch of dried chili flakes
- 840 grams of large russet potatoes
- Pepper and salt to taste
- A drizzle of canola oil
- Half a teaspoon of paprika

Instructions

1. Preheat your oven to 390F.
2. Place a piece of parchment paper on a large tray and set aside.
3. Wash and peel the potatoes, then put them into a spiralizer and run them through until you have several potato curls formed.
4. Put the potato curls onto the tray and leave it there for a couple of minutes so that the parchment paper absorbs the excess moisture, or you can pay them dry.

5. Line a baking tray with pieces of parchment until every surface is covered, then place the now dry potato curls on top, making sure to leave enough space between each curl.
6. Drizzle with oil, then season with Pepper and salt, paprika and chili flakes. Toss lightly, being careful not to break the coils, then place the baking tray into the pre-heated oven.
7. Bake for 20-25 minutes or until the curls are as crisp as you want them to be.
8. Remove and serve hot with a low-FODMAP dip.

NOTE: Remove the fries from the oven every once in a while to remove the ones that are already sufficiently crisped before they burn, then flip the ones that need to be flipped before placing the rest back into the oven.

Low-Fodmap Potato Salad

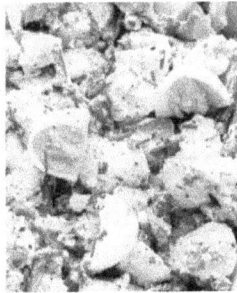

- Prep Time: 20 Minutes
- Cook Time: 25 Minutes
- Yield: 4 Servings
- Calories: 327 Calories
- Nutrition Fact: **Sugars**;6.4g **Proteins**; 13.5g **Fats**; 11.2g **Carbs**;44.4g

What You'll Need

- A quarter teaspoon of black pepper
- 160 grams of green beans

- One(1) tablespoon of lemon juice
- Four(4) large eggs
- A quarter cup of mayonnaise
- One(1) red bell pepper
- Three(3) tablespoons of fresh jives
- One(1) cucumber
- 800 grams of potatoes
- One(1) tablespoon of whole grain mustard
- Three (3) tablespoons of green onions (green part only)

Instructions

1. Wash the potatoes very well, peel them and cut them into bite sized pieces.
2. Cut the green beans into small pieces then set aside.
3. Put the potatoes in a large saucepan, add in enough water to cover the potatoes and set over medium heat and bring to a boil.
4. Cover the saucepan and reduce the heat and allow to simmer for 15-20 minutes or until potatoes are sufficiently tender.
5. 13-17 minutes into simmering the potatoes, add the green beans and cook until the time is over, i.e for about 2-3 minutes or until the green beans are brightly colored and soft.
6. Drain and set aside to cool.
7. Pour some water into a large saucepan, bring it to a boil, then reduce the heat and allow to simmer, then put in the eggs and hard boil them for 10-12 minutes, then remove them and put them into a medium sized bowl, add cold water and set aside to cool.
8. Once the eggs are cool enough to work with, drain them and rinse the eggs under cool water again (as they would have already heated up the water they were kept in, then cut them into quarters.

9. To prepare the bell pepper and cucumber; wash and peel the cucumber, then cut it into short sticks, then deseeded and chop the bell pepper.
10. Finely dice the chives and the green parts of the green onion.
11. To make the salad dressing; out the mayonnaise, lemon juice, a pinch of black pepper and mustard into a medium sized mixing bowl, stir until well combined, preferably with a wooden spoon.
12. Put the eggs, potatoes, bell peppers, green beans, chives, green onions, cucumber and salad dressing into a large mixing bowl, season with a pinch of salt and pepper and stir until well combined.
13. Serve fresh and enjoy!

Low-Fodmap Enchiladas

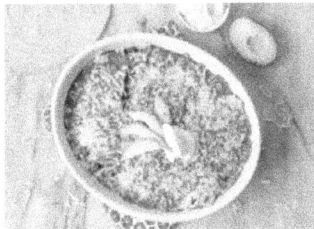

- Prep Time: 40 Minutes
- Cook Time: 20 Minutes
- Yield: 4 Servings
- Calories: 392 Calories
- Nutrition Fact: **Sugars**; 9g **Proteins**; 30g **Fats**; 18g **Carbs**; 23g

What You'll Need

For the enchiladas;

- 200 grams of cheese (grated)
- 350 grams of vegetarian mince or minced beef

- Half a teaspoon of smoked ground paprika
- Two(2) red bell peppers
- Twelve (12) corn tortillas
- Two(2) tablespoons of olive oil

For the sauce;

- Two(2) cups of vegetable broth
- 200 grams of canned diced tomatoes
- Two(2) tablespoons of garlic-infused olive oil
- A pinch of salt
- 70 grams of tomato paste
- A quarter teaspoon of ground cumin
- One (1) tablespoon of cornstarch (to thicken the sauce)
- A quarter teaspoon of oregano
- Two(2) tablespoons of gluten free flour
- Two(2) teaspoons of chilli powder (or less)

For Garnishing;

- Fresh cilantro (optional)
- Avocado (not more that 30 grams per serving)
- Lactose-free sour cream

Instructions

For the sauce;

1. Put two tablespoons of garlic-infused olive oil into a medium sized pan and set it over medium heat.
2. Add the spices and two tablespoons of gluten free flour and stir until well combined.
3. Pour in the vegetable broth, diced tomatoes and tomato paste, stir using a wooden spoon, then cover and allow to boil.
4. Once it is at a rolling boil, resice the heat and allow to simmer for 10-15 minutes more.
5. Add the cornstarch, stir and cook for 3-5 minutes.

For the filling;

1. Pour two tablespoons of olive oil into a large cast iron pan, allow it to heat for a bit on medium-low, n add vegetarian mince.
2. Dice the bell peppers and throw them into the pan, increase the heat to medium and stir fry the minced and bell peppers until fragrant i.e for about 5-8 minutes.
3. Pour in two tablespoons of the sauce into the pan, stir and season with some salt, pepper and ground paprika, then turn off the heat.

For the enchiladas;

1. Preheat your oven to 350F.
2. Pour a few tablespoons of the sauce at the bottom of a medium sized casserole dish.
3. Spread a corn tortilla flat on a clean counter top or flat plate, spread a thin layer of sauce over it, then top with some vegetarian mince and grated cheese.
4. Roll up the tortilla by folding in both edges, then covering that by folding in the sides, then carefully place the wrapped tortilla inside the casserole dish, folded side facing down. Repeat this process until the casserole dish is almost filled, I'd say about ¾ full, i.e if you set them tightly side by side and directly on top of each other.
5. Cover the stacked tortillas with the rest of the enchilada sauce, and top with grated cheese.
6. Carefully place the casserole dish into the oven without jostling it too much, then allow the enchiladas to bake for 20-25 minutes.
7. Remove from the oven when your timer goes off and allow to cool for a few minutes then serve topped with avocados (not more than 30 grams per serving) and lactose-free sour cream and fresh cilantro if you want (I didn't use it).

NOTE: If you find it difficult to wrap up your tortillas, do not despair, it happens to almost every one, even chefs! What you could do thought, is put your tortillas in the casserole dish, fill them and fold them in half and tuck the edges into the dish or at the end of the previously filled tortillas, just be warned that it is going to be pretty messy. Also, if you want the good feel of this Mexican dish, you could try making it spicier by using dutch chilli powder, instead of your regular chilli powder. Since it is a lot spicier, ice recommended at least half a teaspoon, since a teaspoon would be too spicy for a lot of people. Enjoy!

Low-Fodmap Butternut Squash Soup

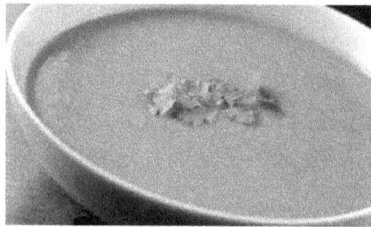

- Prep Time: 15 Minutes
- Cook Time: 75 Minutes
- Yield: 12 Servings
- Calories: 100.6 Calories
- Nutrition Fact: **Sugars**; 4.2g **Proteins**; 1.9g **Fats**;3.0g **Carbs**;19.6g

What You'll Need
- Two(2) cups of water
- Two(2) tablespoons of extra virgin olive oil
- Two(2) cups of almond milk (unsweetened)
- One(1) teaspoon of salt
- 265 grams of carrots (diced)
- Half a teaspoon of black pepper
- 220 grams of celery (diced)

- Half a teaspoon of ground thyme
- 4.2 pounds of butternut squash (cubed)
- Half a teaspoon of rosemary

Instructions

1. Put the oil into a large soup pot and set it over medium heat and allow to simmer for a few seconds, then add the carrots and celery, stir and allow to cook for 10 minutes.
2. Add thyme and rosemary, toss until well combined, then add almond milk, squash, pepper and salt and bring to a rolling boil.
3. Once boiled, set the heat on low and allow to simmer for an hour or more until the vegetables are very soft and fork tender.
4. Remove from heat and blend using an immersion blender or food processor, transfer back to the pot once smooth and adjust seasoning as needed, then cook for a minute more.
5. Serve hot.

NOTE: To get a bit more for, you can switch the water for low-sodium vegetable broth, but in doing so, you will have to reduce the amount of salt in this recipe by half.

Low-Fodmap Pasta

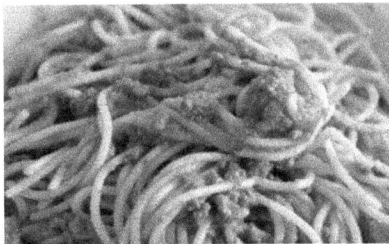

- Prep Time: 15 Minutes
- Cook Time: 60 Minutes
- Yield: 4 Servings

- Calories: 231 Calories
- Nutrition Fact: **Sugars**;6g **Proteins**; 18g **Fats;** 9g **Carbs**; 33g

What You'll Need

- Two(2) tablespoons of parmesan cheese
- Half a pound of ground Beef
- Two(2) cups of rice noodles
- Homemade spaghetti sauce

Instructions

1. Remove the spaghetti sauce from the refrigerator if you haven't and but it in a bowl of warm water (still in the container it was stored in) to unthaw. If it is freshly made, then set it aside until ready for use.
2. Put the ground beef into a pot, add a pinch of salt and half a cup of water, set on low it and allow to simmer for an hour, if there is any water left in it, drain it.
3. Add to the spaghetti sauce and bring to a boil.
4. Boil your pasta until it is a dente, then serve it topped with some ground beef pasta sauce.
5. Dig in!

Low-Fodmap Vegetable Fried Rice

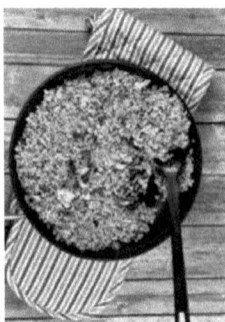

- Prep Time: 10 Minutes
- Cook Time: 12 Minutes
- Yield: 4 Servings
- Calories: 357 Calories
- Nutrition Fact: **Sugars**; 5g **Proteins;** 21g **Fats**; 19g **Carbs**; 32g

What You'll Need

- Two(2) eggs
- Half a cup of carrots (diced)
- Basil or cilantro to garnish
- Three(3) tablespoons of sesame oil
- A quarter cup of tamari
- One tablespoon of lime juice
- Two(2) tablespoons of green onion (diced)
- One(1) cup of spinach
- Half a cup of red peppers (diced)
- Four (4) cups of brown rice (cooked)

Instructions

1. Pour the sesame oil in a large non-stick pan and set it over medium heat until it starts to simmer.
2. Throw in the green onions and sautée for about 3 minutes until fragrant.
3. Add the vegetables and stir fry for a few minutes, then allow to cook for 5 minutes or until vegetables are very tender.
4. Crack the eggs into a bowl, beat them lightly for a few seconds them pour them into the mixture and stir until it begins to scramble.
5. Add tamari and stir until well mixed, then add the cooked rice. Stir using a wooden spoon until well combined, then leave the rice to fry for 3-4 minutes.
6. Add in the lime juice, then stir and turn off the heat.

7. Serve topped with basil or cilantro and enjoy!

Low-Fodmap Lamb And Spinach Curry

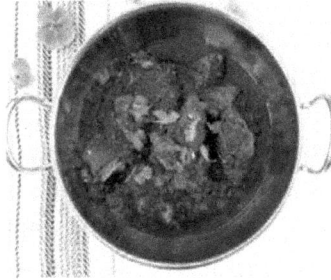

- Prep Time: 20 Minutes
- Cook Time: 60 Minutes
- Yield: 4 Servings
- Calories: 288 Calories
- Nutrition Fact: **Sugars**; 4g **Proteins;** 13g **Fats**; 9g **Carbs**; 11g

What You'll Need

- Pepper and salt to taste
- One(1) teaspoon of turmeric
- 600 grams of diced lamb
- A handful of fresh coriander leaves
- Two(2) tablespoons of garlic flavoured oil
- 200 grams of spinach
- A piece of grated ginger (thumb-size)
- A quarter teaspoon of asafoetida
- 300 grams of fresh tomatoes (roughly grated)
- 5 spring onions (green part only and roughly chopped)
- Two(2) teaspoons of ground cumin
- Two(2) red chillies (deseeded and chopped)
- Two (2) teaspoons of ground coriander

Instructions

1. Put the oil in a medium sized stock bottomed pot, set over medium heat and allow to simmer for a minute or less, then add asafoetida, coriander, cumin and tumeric, stir and cook for a minute or until fragrant.
2. Add the diced lamb and stir until it is fully coated in the cooked mixture, then stir and allow to cook until lightly browned, then add grated tomatoes.
3. Cover the pot with the lid and allow the mixture to simmer over low heat for an hour or until the diced lamb is very tender. Make sure to stir once in a while to make sure it doesn't stick to the bottom of the pot. If it does regardless, add half a cup of water.
4. While the diced lamb cooks, put the spring onions, spinach and coriander into a food processor and blitz it until it is smooth. If you do not have a food processor, does slice them thinly by hand.
5. Add the vegetable paste into the lamb mix, stir until well combined, then allow to cook for a few more minutes or until it is at a rolling boil.
6. Season with Pepper and salt as needed.
7. Add a little red chilli, then serve with steamed rice.

Low-Fodmap Kale Salad

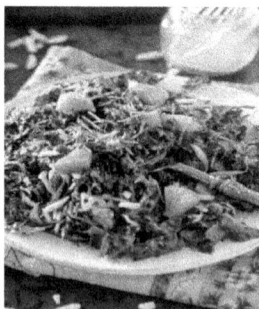

- Prep Time: 22 Minutes

- Cook Time: 3 Minutes
- Yield: 8 Servings
- Calories: 145 Calories
- Nutrition Fact: **Sugars**; 8g **Proteins**; 4g **Fats**; 9g **Carbs**; 16g

What You'll Need

- 70 grams of dried cranberries
- A quarter teaspoon of kosher salt
- Three(3) tablespoons of extra virgin olive oil
- Half a cup of slightly toasted sliced almonds
- One (1) tablespoon of freshly squeezed lemon juice
- One(1) tablespoon of mustard
- One(1) orange
- 455 grams of curly kale (washed, stemmed and cut into pieces)
- One(1) tablespoon of Sherry vinegar
- A quarter teaspoon of freshly ground black pepper
- Four(4) medium sized carrots (scrubbed or peeled)

Instructions

For the dressing;

1. Put the lemon juice, mustard, olive oil and vinegar into a small mixing bowl and stir to combine. Once well combined, season with pepper and salt to taste, then set aside.

For the salad;

1. Cut and peel the orange, remove the veins and seeds and release the segments into a medium sized bowl, then set aside also.
2. Fit your food processor with the metal blade and put the kale inside it in batches until they are all chopped, remove the kale and set it aside, then exchange the blade in a food processor for a shredding disk, put in carrots and process until they are well shredded, then add them to the chopped kale.

71

3. Put the cranberries and almonds into the kale mixture, stir until well combined, then slowly fold in the dressing into it is fully incorporated.
4. Serve immediately or store in an airtight jar for up to four days.

NOTE: If you do not have a food processor, you have no need to worry, just wash the kale properly, then dump it in a large bowl, wash your hands and get to work! All you need to do is give the kale a good massage. No jokes! Just knead the kale, put some muscle into it, use your knuckles and you will have a couple of relaxed kale leaves on your hands. Literally! What this massage does is to reduce the fibrous texture of the leaves and makes it very easy for you to slice. They don't have to be as thin as a thread, but try to slice them as finely as you can and you can

Chapter Nine: Low-Fodmap Dinner Recipes

Who says you can't have dinner fit for a king? Your food options are not limited, they are just modified. So, bear that in mind as you make the most delicious Low-FODMAP dinner ever! You'll have your friends and family wishing they had IBS too...or not.

Low-Fodmap Chicken And Rice

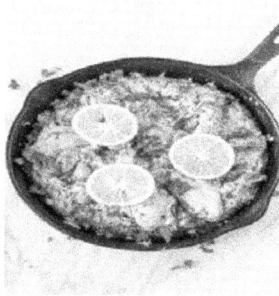

- Prep Time: 10 Minutes
- Cook Time: 22 Minutes
- Yield: 4 Servings
- Calories: 433 calories
- Nutrition Fact: **Sugars**; 6.2g **Proteins**; 33.6g **Fats**; 13.9g **Carbs**; 41.9g

What You'll Need

- Two(2) cups of Low-FODMAP chicken broth
- Parsley (optional)
- Two(2) tablespoons of garlic-infused olive oil
- Two(2) tablespoons of Low-FODMAP Italian seasoning
- One(1) tablespoon of freshly squeezed lemon juice
- One(1) pack of boneless, skinless chicken thighs

- One(1) cup of uncooked white rice

Instructions

1. Pour the olive oil into a large skillet and set over medium heat, allow to simmer for a few seconds.
2. Add the chicken thigh and fry for 2 minutes on each side until lightly browned, remove from pan and set aside.
3. Add the rice to the hot pan, then stir in lemon juice, chicken broth and Italian seasoning. Stir well until fully combined.
4. Put the chicken on top of the rice and cook covered for 20 minutes over medium heat or until the liquid in the rice is completely absorbed.
5. Serve garnished with parsley.

NOTE: If your stove burns bright, you might want to cook the rice on low so that your rice doesn't burn. You should also avoid stirring the rice before the liquid in it is fully absorbed if not it will burn. If you must stir, do not stir deeply, just put the spoon or spatula until it gets to the middle, scoop some rice and turn it upside down, repeat this process until you have turned the whole top of the rice.

Low-Fodmap Sour Chicken Rice

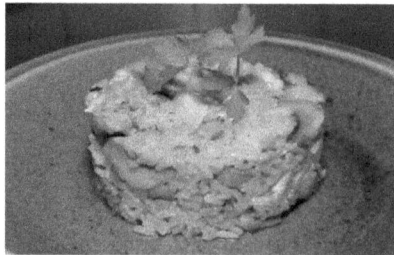

- Prep Time: 20 Minutes
- Cook Time:15 Minutes
- Yield: 3 Servings

- Calories: 251 Calories
- Nutrition Fact: **Sugars**; 3g **Proteins**; 14.3 **Fats**; 13.7g **Carbs**; 22g

What You'll Need

- Two(2) tablespoons of fresh chives
- Two(2) finely sliced chicken breasts
- One(1) tablespoon of white rice vinegar
- Two(2) tablespoons of garlic-infused oil
- Two(2) tablespoons of Low-FODMAP ketchup
- Two(2) tablespoons of sugar
- Two(2) tablespoons of pineapple juice
- Two(2) rings of pineapple (diced)
- One(1) tablespoon of corn flour (mixed with two tablespoons of water to make a paste)
- Half a piece of green pepper (diced)
- Two(2) cups of cooked white rice

Instructions

1. Put one tablespoon of garlic-infused olive oil into a large pan, throw in the green peppers and fry them until they are slightly browned.
2. Put the white rice, Low-FODMAP ketchup, pineapple juice, vinegar and sugar into a large mixing bowl, stir until well combined, then add it to the fried green peppers, then cook over high heat for 5-10 minutes.
3. Add the corn flour paste, stir until well mixed then add the diced pineapples and chopped chicken breasts, stir and cook for 3 minutes.
4. Cut the chives into tiny bits and sprinkle it over the rice and cook covered for another minute.
5. Set aside to cool for a while, then serve, or you could put them in plastic containers and refrigerate. All you need to do when you are ready to eat, is microwave, then you are good to go!

Low-Fodmap Chicken Curry

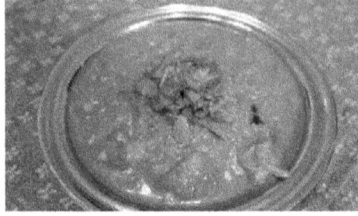

- Prep Time: 10 Minutes
- Cook Time: 25 Minutes
- Yield: 3 Servings
- Calories: 290 Calories
- Nutrition Fact: **Sugars**; 3g **Proteins**; 27g **Fats**; 12g **Carbs**; 10g

What You'll Need

- A quarter teaspoon of salt
- Two(2) finely sliced chicken breast
- A handful of spinach
- 300 grams of chopped tomatoes
- One (1) tablespoon of basil puree
- Two(2) tablespoons of mixed herbs
- A pinch of black pepper
- One (1) tablespoon of garlic-infused olive oil

Instructions

1. Put the oil into a large saucepan and allow to simmer for 30 seconds-1 minute,a few seconds, then add the chopped chicken breast and fry until they are seared.
2. Put in the chopped tomatoes, then add the basil puree, salt and pepper to taste and mixed herbs, stir until well combined.

3. Add the spinach, stir and allow to cook until wilted.
4. Allow to cool, then serve into bowls and enjoy!

Low-Fodmap Leek And Potato Soup

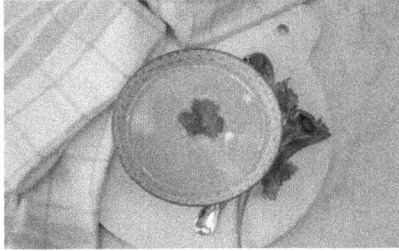

- Prep Time: 10 Minutes
- Cook Time: 25 Minutes
- Yield: 4 Servings
- Calories: 196 Calories
- Nutrition Fact: **Sugars**; 7g **Proteins**; 18g **Fats;** 8g **Carbs**; 16g

What You'll Need

- A quarter teaspoon of freshly ground pepper
- One(1) cup of thinly sliced leeks (green part only)
- Two(2) cups of lactose free whole milk
- Three(3) medium yellow potatoes (peeled and diced)
- Two(2) tablespoons fresh parsley
- One(1) tablespoon of unsalted butter
- Two(2) cups of Low-FODMAP Vegetable broth

Instructions

1. Put the butter into a large saucepan and leave to melt, then add the leaks and cook over medium-low heat for 10 minutes.
2. Pour in a cup of vegetable broth and bring to a rolling boil i.e about 2-3 minutes.

3. Add the rest of the broth, potatoes and parsley to pan, stir and allow to simmer on low heat for about 20 minutes or until potatoes are very tender.
4. Let the cooked vegetables cool for a while, then blend it with an immersion blender, add the milk and stir until fully combined.
5. Serve topped with some cilantro and enjoy!

Low-Fodmap Tomato Soup

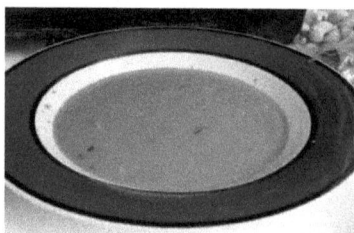

- Prep Time: 10 Minutes
- Cook Time: 15 Minutes
- Yield: 4 Servings
- Calories: 247 Calories
- Nutrition Fact: **Sugars**; 8g **Proteins**; 15g **Fats**; 12g **Carbs**; 6g

What You'll Need

- One(1) tablespoon of fresh basil (minced)
- Three(3) tablespoons of olive oil
- Pepper and salt to taste
- Half an onion (roughly chopped)
- A cup of diced tomatoes
- A quarter cup of whipping cream
- Three(3) tablespoons of tomato paste
- One(1) cup of Low-FODMAP chicken broth

Instructions

1. Pour olive oil into a small frying pan and set it over medium heat, until it is thoroughly heated, then add the onions and stir fry for 3-5 minutes until they are browned and fragrant.
2. Use a cheesecloth to strain the oil into a medium sized saucepan.
3. Heat the onion infused olive oil over low heat and add the diced tomatoes, stir and allow to cook for 2 minutes or until the tomatoes lose all moisture, then add chicken broth, tomato paste and pepper and salt to taste.
4. Bring to a rolling boil, then reduce the heat and allow to simmer for five minutes.
5. Remove the saucepan from heat and blend the mixture smooth using an immersion blender.
6. Add fresh basil and whipping cream, stir and serve immediately.

Low-Fodmap Vegetable Soup

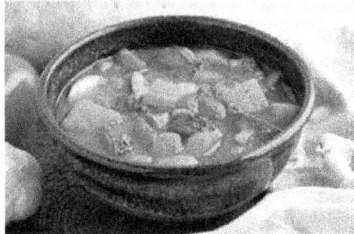

- Prep Time: 15 Minutes
- Cook Time: 30 Minutes
- Yield: 8 Servings
- Calories: 340 Calories
- Nutrition Fact: **Sugars**; 9g **Proteins**; 22g **Fats**; 11g **Carbs**; 17g

What You'll Need

- A quarter teaspoon of kosher salt
- A quarter cup of olive oil
- Eight(8) cups of Low-FODMAP Vegetable broth
- 85 grams of rind of parmesan cheese
- Two (2) cloves of garlic (peeled)
- One(1) medium zucchini (cut into bite-sized pieces)
- One(1) cup of finely sliced leeks (green parts only)
- 55 grams of kale (hard stems removed and torn into bite sized pieces)
- A quarter cup of finely sliced scallions (green parts only)
- 455 grams of red potatoes (washed and cut into bite-sized pieces)
- One(1) cup of yellow corn kernels
- 170 grams of green beans (diced)
- Two(2) medium carrots (peeled and cut into bite-sized pieces)
- Half a piece of fennel bulb (stalks and fronds discarded, cut into bite-sized pieces)
- 340 grams of plum tomatoes (cored and chopped)
- A quarter teaspoon of freshly ground black pepper

Instructions

1. Put the oil into a medium sized stock pot and set over medium-low heat, then allow to simmer for a minute or less, until well heated.
2. Throw in the garlic and saute for a minute or two until soft but not browned, then use a perforated spoon or spatula to remove all the pieces of garlic (this makes the recipe Low-FODMAP).
3. Once you have removed all the garlic, add the scallions and leeks, stir and cook for 3 minutes or until softened.
4. Pour in the broth and stir, then add the carrots and potatoes then allow to simmer for 2 minutes.
5. Cover with a lid and allow to simmer for another 13 minutes or until the carrots and potatoes are fork tender.

6. Add the zucchini, tomatoes, kale, beans, cheese rind and fennel, stir and allow to simmer for 25 minutes.
7. Season with pepper and salt.
8. Serve into bowls or put into airtight containers and refrigerate for as long as four months.

NOTE: You can also use garlic infused olive oil in lieu of the regular olive oil.

Low-Fodmap Beef Bourguignon

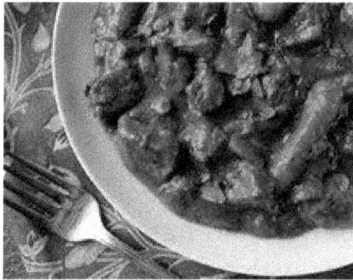

- Prep Time: 20 Minutes
- Cook Time: 16 Minutes
- Yield: 6 Servings
- Calories: 330 Calories
- Nutrition Fact: Sugars;2g Proteins;34g Fats; 11g Carbs; 15g

What You'll Need
- Half a teaspoon of black pepper
- Half a cup of arrowroot flour
- Half a cup of fresh parsley (chopped)
- Half a cup of beef bone broth
- Two(2) whole bay leaves (dried)
- Two (2) tablespoons of tomato paste

- Four (4) medium green onions (chopped and green part only)
- One (1) teaspoon of sea salt
- One (1) cup of diced carrots
- Half a teaspoon of dried thyme
- A cup of red wine
- Two (2) pounds of stewed beef
- Two (2) tablespoons of olive oil

Instructions

1. Put the arrowroot flour into a bowl, add pepper and salt, then stir until well combined. Add the meat and stir by hand or use a wooden ladle until the meat is evenly coated in the flour mixture.
2. Pour some of the marinated meat into zip-lock bags or quart freezer bags.
3. Share an even amount of the rest of the ingredients between the ziplock- bags or the quart freezer bags.
4. Tag each of the bags with a paper tape and label them, then set them in a refrigerator.
5. When ready to serve; the first thing you need to do is thaw the soup. So pour the oil into a large cast iron pan and set over medium heat, allow to simmer for 30 seconds, then add the beef and allow to fry until both sides are seared.
6. Then, gently remove the beef from the pan and put it in a slow cooker .
7. Pour half a cup of red one into the pan to deglaze it.
8. Throw the vegetables into the slow cooker and pour the redwine from the pan over it, then stir to make sure that the ingredients are evenly distributed.
9. Cook covered on low for a total of 4-6 hours.
10. Remove the bayleaves, then serve.

Chapter Ten: Soups, Vegetables, And Salads

Here are the stars of a full course meal and you can have your pick without worrying about any abdominal discomfort or bloating. With these celebrities, you can say goodbye to flatulence and mean it! These recipes are sure to give you the relief you've been searching for. So, dig in!

Low-Fodmap Corn Salad

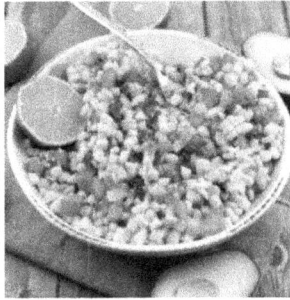

- Prep Time: 10 Minutes
- Cook Time: 10 Minutes
- Yield: 6 Servings
- Calories: 200 Calories
- Nutrition Facts: **Sugars**; 8g **Proteins**; 11g **Fats**; 5g **Carbs**; 19g

What You'll Need

- A quarter cup of Low-FODMAP salsa
- Four (4) corns on the corn
- A quarter cup of fresh cilantro (roughly chopped)
- One(1) medium sized tomato (chopped)
- Half a tablespoon of lime juice

Instructions

1. Put some water into a large stock bottomed pot, add a pinch or two of salt, then put in the corns and bring to boil, then continue cooking on high for 5 minutes.
2. Remove the corns from the water and carefully remove the kernels from the cob and put them into a bowl.
3. Add the tomatoes, salsa, cilantro and lime juice.
4. Stir until well combined, then serve and enjoy!

Low-Fodmap Spinach And Blueberry Salad

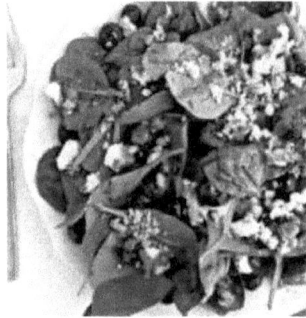

- Prep Time: 10 Minutes
- Cook Time: 0 Minutes
- Yield: 4 Servings
- Calories: 142 Calories
- Nutrition Facts: **Sugars**; 3g **Proteins**; 17g **Fats**; 11g **Carbs**; 7g

What You'll Need

- Half a cup of feta cheese
- Eight (8) cups of baby spinach
- Half a cup of chopped walnuts
- One(1) cup of fresh blueberries

For the dressing;

- A pinch of pepper
- A quarter cup of fresh blueberries
- Half a tablespoon of sugar

- A quarter cup of olive oil
- A pinch of salt
- A quarter cup of red wine vinegar

Instructions

1. Put the feta cheese, blueberries, spinach and walnuts into a bowl and toss until well combined, then serve them into four serving bowls.
2. Put all the ingredients for the dressing into a blender, pulse until smooth, then pour the dressing over the served bowls of salads.

Low-Fodmap Chicken Soup

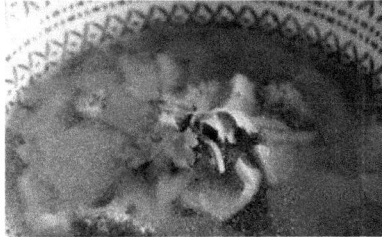

- Prep Time: 10 Minutes
- Cook Time: 15 Minutes
- Yield: 3 Servings
- Calories: 228 Calories
- Nutrition Facts: **Sugars**; 5g **Proteins**; 24g **Fats**; 9g **Carbs**; 12g

What You'll Need

- Half a piece of white potato (peeled and cut into squares)
- Four(4) cups of organic chicken broth
- Three(3) sprigs of cilantro
- One(1) tablespoons of coconut oil
- One(1) zucchini (peeled and cut into squares)
- Three(3) cups of water
- One(1) chicken breast (sliced)
- Half a cup of broccoli

- Half a tablespoon of tamari
- One(1) carrot (peeled and chopped)
- Half a teaspoon of white Pepper

Instructions

1. Put the coconut oil, broth, pepper, water, and tamari into a medium sized saucepan, set it over medium heat and bring to a boil, then reduce and allow to simmer on low for 20 minutes.
2. Put in the chicken and cook for another 2 minutes.
3. Throw in the vegetables and cook for 5 minutes.
4. Serve topped with a sprig of cilantro and enjoy!

Low-Fodmap Carrot Soup

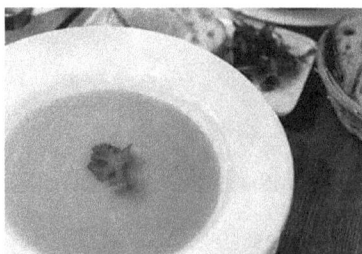

- Prep Time: 5 Minutes
- Cook Time: 20 Minutes
- Yield: 3 Servings
- Calories: 265 Calories
- Nutrition Facts: **Sugars**; 6g **Proteins**; 21g **Fats**; 14g **Carbs**; 16g

What You'll Need

- One(1) bayleaf
- One(1) teaspoon of oregano
- Two(2) tablespoons of grated Parmesan cheese
- Two(2) teaspoons of ginger
- Two(2) cups of Low-FODMAP Vegetable broth

- Two(2) tablespoons of olive oil
- One(1) teaspoon of salt
- 450 grams of carrots (peeled and chopped)
- 680 grams of tomatoes

Instructions

1. Pour the oil into a sauce pan and set over medium heat, once it's heated, add the carrots and ginger, stir fry for a minute or until fragrant.
2. Add the oregano, tomatoes and salt, stir, then add the cheese, broth and bayleaf, stir to combine, then bring to a boil.
3. Reduce the heat and allow to simmer for 15-20 minutes or until the carrots are soft.
4. Turn off the heat and remove bay leaves, then use an immersion blender to puree the mixture.
5. Season with Pepper and salt to taste.
6. Serve.

Low-Fodmap Potato Soup

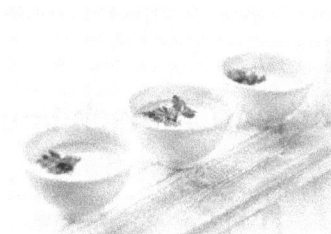

- Prep Time: 10 Minutes
- Cook Time: 30 Minutes
- Yield: 4 Servings
- Calories: 750 Calories
- Nutrition Facts: **Sugars**; 20g **Proteins**; 35g **Fats**; 38g **Carbs**; 71g

What You'll Need

- Two(2) green onions (green part only and sliced)
- Six(6) medium sized russet potatoes (peeled and chopped)
- A quarter cup of grated Parmesan cheese
- Six (6) cups of lactose-free milk
- A quarter cup of butter
- Half a cup of gluten free flour
- A quarter teaspoon of cracked black pepper
- A pinch of salt

Instructions

1. Boil the potatoes for about 15 minutes or until they are fork-tender, drain and blend it until smooth in a food processor.
2. Melt the butter in a large saucepan, then add the flour and cook for a minute, stirring continuously so that it doesn't stick.
3. Pour in three cups of milk with a pinch of salt and pepper, then stir using a wooden ladle until all the lumps dissolve. Add the potato paste and the remaining milk, bring to a rolling boil, stirring every once in a while.
4. Turn of the heat and add the cheese and one green onion, stir until the cheese melts, then serve topped with the rest of the onion.

Low-Fodmap Spinach Soup

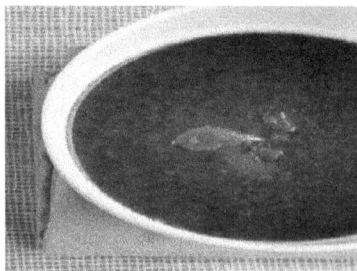

- Prep Time: 10 Minutes
- Cook Time: 10 Minutes
- Yield: 3 Servings
- Calories: 327 Calories
- Nutrition Facts: **Sugars**; 2g **Proteins**; 17g **Fats**; 8g **Carbs**; 4g

What You'll Need

- Two(2) cups of water
- 180 grams of Low-FODMAP coconut milk
- One(1) teaspoon of curry powder
- One(1) tablespoon of olive oil
- 225 grams of fresh spinach
- Half a teaspoon of turmeric
- One(1) leek (only green part)
- One(1) courgette
- Half a teaspoon of cumin
- 8 grams of Low-FODMAP stock cube

Instructions

1. Dice the courgettes and put the water into the kettle and set it over medium heat and bring it to a boil.
2. Pour the oil into a pan and heat it over medium heat, add the spices and sautée for a minute or two.
3. Throw in the courgettes and leeks, stir and cook until soft then add the boiled water and stock cube.
4. Bring to a boil, then reduce the heat and allow to simmer for a little over 5 minutes.
5. Add the spinach and coconut milk and allow to boil again, then cook on low until the spinach softens.
6. Serve!

Low-Fodmap Roasted Vegetables

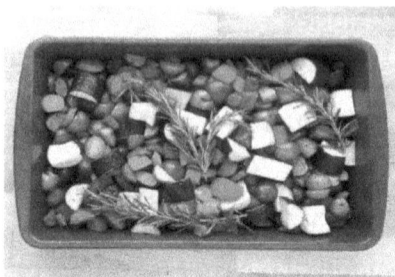

- Prep Time: 15 Minutes
- Cook Time: 90 Minutes
- Yield: 6 Servings
- Calories: 290 Calories
- Nutrition Facts: **Sugars**; 5.3g **Proteins**; 2.7g **Fats**; 9.6g **Carbs**; 24.9g

What You'll Need

- A quarter cup of garlic infused olive oil
- Three(3) medium carrots (cut into bite-sized pieces)
- One(1) small rutabaga (peeled and cut into bite-sized pieces)
- Two(2) medium parsnips (peeled and cut into bite-sized pieces
- Two(2) medium-sized Yukon gold potatoes
- Pepper and salt to taste

Instructions

1. Preheat your oven to 375F.
2. Put the vegetables into a large bowl add the oil and toss until they are well coated.
3. Put the vegetables on a baking sheet and sprinkle with pepper and salt.
4. Bake for 45 minutes or until the vegetables are lightly browned.

5. Serve warm.

Low-Fodmap Vegetable Chilli

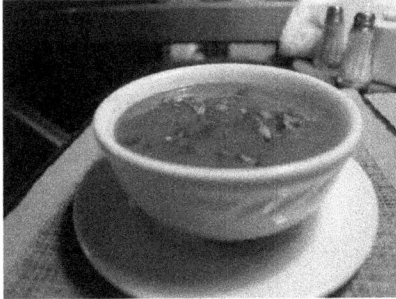

- Prep Time: 10 Minutes
- Cook Time: 30 Minutes
- Yield: 4 Servings
- Calories: 309 Calories
- Nutrition Facts: **Sugars**; 4g **Proteins**; 28g **Fats**; 15g **Carbs**; 21g

What You'll Need

- A handful of chopped coriander
- One(1) red chilli (deseeded and chopped)
- One(1) tablespoon of garlic infused olive oil
- A handful of chives
- Two(2) courgettes (chopped)
- One(1) can of crushed tomatoes
- 100 grams of quinoa (washed and drained)
- One(1) can of chickpeas (drained and rinsed)
- One(1) small cinnamon sticks
- Two(2) teaspoons of ground cumin
- Half a cup of water
- Two(2) carrots (peeled and chopped)
- One(1) red pepper (chopped)
- One(1) teaspoon of cayenne pepper

Instructions

1. Put the oil into a medium sized pan and set over medium heat, allow to simmer for a few seconds, then add the peppers, chilli and courgettes.
2. Add the chickpeas, crushed tomatoes, quinoa and water, stir and bring to a boil, then reduce the heat and allow to simmer for 20 minutes or until the quinoa is à dente.
3. Add the coriander and chives, stir and cook for 2 more minutes, then serve.

Low-Fodmap Vegetable Burger

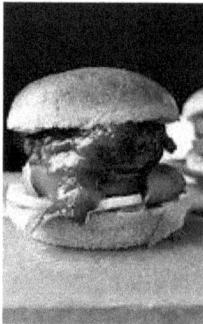

- Prep Time: 10 Minutes
- Cook Time: 20 Minutes
- Yield: 4 Servings
- Calories: 174 Calories
- Nutrition Facts: **Sugars**;5g **Proteins**; 18g **Fats**; 11g **Carbs**; 23g

What You'll Need

- 20 grams of coriander
- Half a teaspoon of smoked paprika
- 30 grams of sunflower seeds
- Pepper and salt to taste

- 140 grams of canned butter beans (rinsed and drained)
- One(1) slice of gluten free bread
- 50 grams of walnuts
- Three(3) tablespoons of olive oil
- Half a teaspoon of chilli flakes
- 200 grams of brown rice
- Two(2) spring onions (green part only)
- One(1) tablespoon of sesame seeds

Instructions

1. The first thing to do is cook your rice then set aside.
2. Put the butter beans into a small bowl and mash them lightly with a fork until they have small lumps in them.
3. Set a small skillet over medium heat , allow to heat up for a few seconds then add the raw walnuts, toast them until they are lightly browned i.e for about 5-7 minutes. Set aside to cool for a bit.
4. Cut the spring onions and coriander into small bits, then add it to the bowl of mashed beans.
5. Once the walnuts are cool enough, chop them into bits and add them to the bowl of mashed beans and vegetables.
6. Add the cooked rice (make sure it doesn't contain any water), sunflower and sesame seeds, oil, salt and all the spices.
7. Mix everything properly by hand or use a wooden ladle if you will be bothered by the mess.
8. Share the mixture into four places, then form your patties.
9. If you are using a grill, lightly brush the grill with some oil, then allow it to heat for a bit. If you do not have a grill, then you can use the skillet used to toast the walnuts, heat it up over medium-low heat.
10. Once heated, add a small amount of oil (enough to coat the bottom of the pan), then add your burgers, or put the burgers in the grill and close the lid.
11. Cook on each side for 4-5 minutes until well browned. If the heat seems too high, then reduce it.

12. Remove the burgers from heat and set aside to cool for a bit, they won't be as firm as your regular burger but they will hold fine.
13. While the burgers cool, prepare your toppings and sides, also don't forget to toast your buns a bit.
14. Serve as you would a regular burger and enjoy!

Chapter Eleven: Appetizers

If you are looking for a few little somethings to wet your appetite, then you are at the right place! Nah...don't worry about that, they are all perfectly safe for people with IBS. I'd say they were specially made for them, I mean, who else can really enjoy these Low-FODMAP Recipes? Don't answer that, just jump right in!

Low-Fodmap Tomato Bruschetta

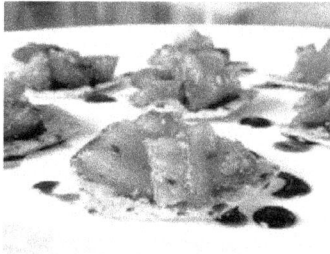

- Prep Time: 5 Minutes
- Cook Time: 5 Minutes
- Yield: 3 Servings
- Calories: 130 Calories
- Nutrition Facts: **Sugars**; 2g **Proteins**; 7g **Fats**; 6g **Carbs**; 19g

What You'll Need

- One(1) teaspoon of dried basil
- One(1) teaspoon of balsamic reduction
- Half a teaspoon of dried parsley
- Three(3) medium tomatoes
- One(1) teaspoon of dried chives
- Two(2) tablespoons of extra virgin olive oil
- A pinch of sea salt
- Two(2) teaspoons of balsamic vinegar
- Half a teaspoon of dried oregano

Instructions

1. To begin, rinse your tomatoes with tepid water, deseeded, then chop them.
2. Put the tomatoes into a medium sized mixing bowl, then add the vinegar, spices, reduction, and olive oil, stir to combine, then season with salt (more if needed). Set aside to marinate for 30 minutes.
3. Serve with crackers or baguettes with a drizzle of balsamic reduction.

Low-Fodmap Spring Rolls

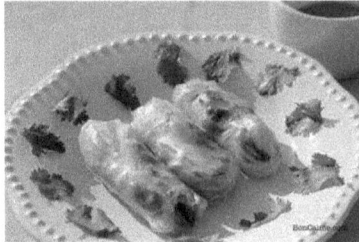

- Prep Time: 15 Minutes
- Cook Time: 40 Minutes
- Yield: 5 Servings
- Calories: 279 Calories
- Nutrition Facts: **Sugars**; 2g **Proteins**; 24g **Fats**; 8g **Carbs**; 12g

What You'll Need

Filling;

- One(1) carrot
- Rice paper
- Half a cup of basil
- One(1) turnip
- One(1) cup of cilantro
- Twelve(12) medium-sized shrimps

- Half a cup of mint
- One(1) zucchini

Marinate;

- A pinch of white Pepper
- Two(2) teaspoons of chopped ginger
- One(1) tablespoon of garlic infused olive oil
- One(1) tablespoon of scallions (green part only)
- One(1) teaspoon of fish sauce
- One(1) tablespoon of coconut oil
- Two(2) teaspoons of gluten free soy sauce

Peanut Sauce;

- Two(2) tablespoons of wheat free soy sauce
- A quarter cup of natural smooth peanut butter (sugar free)
- Two(2) teaspoons of fish sauce
- Two(2) tablespoons of freshly squeezed lime juice
- Two(2) teaspoons of natural cane syrup
- One(1) teaspoon of dried chilli flakes
- Two(2) tablespoons of garlic infused olive oil

Instructions

To marinate the shrimp;

1. Put all the marinade ingredients into a ziplock bag, add the shrimps (make sure they are fully covered) then refrigerate for a little over 30 minutes.
2. Put all the peanut sauce ingredients into a large mixing bowl, stir with a wooden ladle until well combined.
3. Cut up or julienne the turnip, carrot and zucchini.
4. Put the coconut oil into a large skillet and saute all the ingredients (except mint and basil leaves) for the following for 1-2 minutes (do not overcook).
5. To make the spring rolls; Dip the rice paper into a large bowl of water for 3-5 seconds until it softens a bit, then remove it and a bit of all the vegetables, cilantro and shrimp, then break the mint leaves and basil by hand and put them in the rolls.

6. Fold in the sides, then gently roll the wraps and voila! Your very own Low-FODMAP spring rolls!

NOTE: You really have to work fast with the rice paper as they get really sticky when wet and tend to break apart as they lose moisture. So, tick tick goes the clock!

Low-Fodmap Cheese Bread

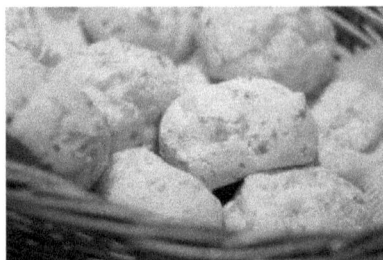

- Prep Time: 12 Minutes
- Cook Time: 30 Minutes
- Yield: 8 Servings
- Calories: 160 Calories
- Nutrition Facts: **Sugars**; 7g **Proteins**; 19g **Fats**; 13.7g **Carbs**; 16.3g

What You'll Need

- One(1) teaspoon of sea salt
- One(1) cup of lactose free milk
- Two(2) eggs
- One(1) cup of parmesan cheese
- Half a cup of coconut oil
- Two(2) cups of tapioca Flour

Instructions

1. Preheat your oven to 450F.
2. Pour the milk into a medium-sized saucepan, set over medium heat and bring to a slow boil. Once bubbles start to form at the top of the milk, remove from heat.

3. Pour the tapioca flour into the milk, stir using a wooden ladle until all the flour is incorporated and no lumps are formed and the mixture starts to thicken like gelatin, then set aside to cool for a bit.
4. Beat the dough for a couple of minutes at medium speed using a standing mixer fitted with a paddle attachment.
5. Crack the egg into a small bowl and whisk until foamy, then slowly fold them into the dough, make sure to scrape down the sides of the bowl.
6. Add the cheese and beat until fully incorporated and your dough is stretchy, soft and sticky.
7. Line a baking sheet with parchment paper, then scoop some dough into it using an ice cream scoop.
8. Coat your hands or ice cream scoop with some olive oil if the dough gets too sticky to work with.
9. Place the baking sheet into the preheated oven and allow the dough to bake for 25-30 minutes.
10. Remove from the oven once the top of the bread appears dry and starts to show orange flecks of color.

Low-Fodmap Cucumber Bites

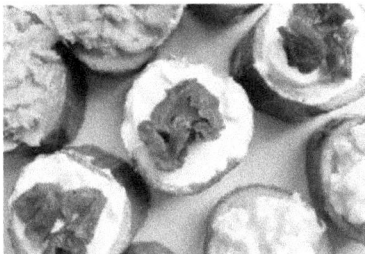

- Prep Time: 30 Minutes
- Cook Time: 0 Minutes
- Yield: 20 Servings

- Calories: 159 Calories
- Nutrition Facts: **Sugars**; 2.1g **Proteins**; 11.9g **Fats**; 9g **Carbs**; 4g

What You'll Need

- One(1) tablespoon of roasted paprika
- Half a cup of lactose-free cream cheese
- Two(2) cucumbers
- Half a cup of Low-FODMAP egg salad
- Half a cup of Low-FODMAP tuna salad

Instructions

1. Chop the cucumbers into round bite-sized pieces, then use a spoon to make a small groove in the middle.
2. Scoop some egg salad over a third of the cucumber slices, then the tuna salad over another third and the cream cheese over the rest, taking care not to over top them lest they start to fall off.
3. Drain and cut the roasted paprika into small pieces, then top the cream cheese with the roasted paprika and serve.

Low-Fodmap Salmon Cakes

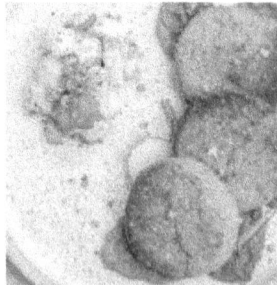

- Prep Time: 10 Minutes
- Cook Time: 40 Minutes
- Yield: 2 Servings
- Calories: 226 Calories

- Nutrition Facts: **Sugars**; 3g **Proteins**; 6.5g **Fats**; 13.8g **Carbs**; 25g

What You'll Need

- Pepper and salt to taste
- Half a tablespoon of coconut flour
- Two(2) medium carrots
- One(1) lemon zest
- A handful of chives (chopped)
- A can of wild salmon
- Half a tablespoon of coconut oil

Instructions

1. Preheat your oven to 400F.
2. Line a baking sheet with pieces of parchment paper.
3. Peel and chop the carrots, then put them into a food processor, pulse until the carrots are small and well diced up.
4. Open the can of salmons and drain it of all liquid, then set aside.
5. Add the rest of the ingredients into the food processor, along with the salmons, pulse until well combined and almost smooth.
6. Use your hand to form the mixture into palm-sized cakes, using a paper towel to pat any excess liquid.
7. Gently place the newly formed cakes onto your baking sheet and place them in the oven.
8. Bake for 40 minutes or more if you want them a bit crispy.
9. Serve warm.

Low-Fodmap Pizza Bites

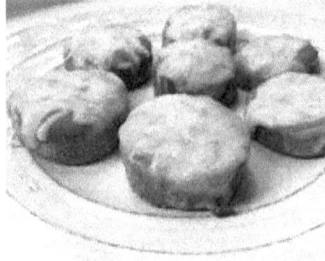

- Prep Time: 5 Minutes
- Cook Time: 5 Minutes
- Yield: 4 Servings
- Calories: 231 Calories
- Nutrition Facts: **Sugars**;2g **Proteins**; 4g **Fats**; 3g **Carbs**; 7g

What You'll Need

- Pepper and salt to taste
- Two(2) large zucchini (sliced)
- A quarter cup of Mozzarella (shredded)
- A quarter cup of Low-FODMAP sauce
- A quarter cup of tomatoes (sliced)
- About half a teaspoon of Italian seasoning (for sprinkling)

Instructions

1. Line a baking sheet with pieces of parchment paper.
2. Put the sliced zucchini onto the pre-lined baking sheet, then place the baking sheet into the oven and broil for 2 minutes on each side.
3. Top with the rest of the ingredients, then broil for 3 more minutes or until the cheese is completely melted, then remove from the oven and sprinkle the Italian seasoning over it.

Low-Fodmap Shrimp Ceviche

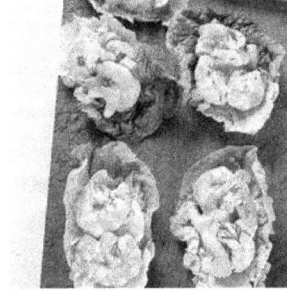

- Prep Time: 10 Minutes
- Cook Time: 20 Minutes
- Yield: 3 Servings
- Calories: 307 Calories
- Nutrition Facts: **Sugars**; 3.1g **Proteins**; 19.6g **Fats**; 14.7g **Carbs**; 13.8g

What You'll Need

- A pinch of black pepper
- One(1) ripe avocado (diced)
- A quarter teaspoon of kosher salt
- Some Low-FODMAP sauce for serving
- A pound of shrimp (peeled and deveined)
- One(1) head of butter lettuce (leaves removed and separated)
- Half a tablespoon of garlic infused olive oil
- One(1) small cucumber (diced)
- Half a tablespoon of freshly squeezed lemon juice
- One(1) tablespoon of fresh cilantro (chopped)

Instructions

1. Put a few pinches of salt into a pot of water, set over medium heat and bring to a boil, add the shrimps into the

pot of boiling water and cook for a little over a minute or until the shrimp are almost pink.
2. Drain the shrimp and rinse under cold running water.
3. Chop the shrimp into bite-sized pieces and put them into a medium sized mixing bowl.
4. Add the rest of the ingredients into the bowl of shrimps and stir until well combined.
5. Refrigerate for an hour, then scoop up the ceviche into the lettuce leaves and serve topped with some Low-FODMAP sauce.

Low-Fodmap Eggplant Stack

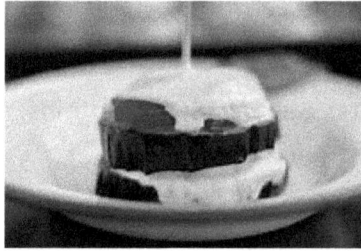

- Prep Time: 20 Minutes
- Cook Time: 25 Minutes
- Yield: 4 Servings
- Calories: 155 Calories
- Nutrition Facts: **Sugars**; 1g **Proteins**; 8g **Fats**; 10g **Carbs**; 11g

What You'll Need

- Half a cup of Mozzarella cheese
- A pound of fresh eggplant (unpeeled)
- A pinch of salt
- Half a cup of fresh basil
- One(1) tablespoon of garlic infused olive oil
- A pinch of freshly ground black pepper
- Half a jar of roasted red peppers (drained and rinsed)
- One(1) medium tomato

Instructions

1. First of all, preheat your broiler.
2. Cut the eggplant in circles until you have four even size pairs (keep the rest for later use), then coat them lightly on both sides with garlic-infused oil, then season with pepper and salt.
3. Line a baking sheet with pieces of parchment, then place the eggplants onto baking sheet, then put them into the broiler and set your timer for 4 minutes or broil on each side for 3-4 minutes until the eggplants are golden brown.
4. Remove the baking sheet and set the oven to 425F.
5. Dice the bell pepper and cut the tomato into rounds, also cut the cheese into thin slices.
6. Then top the cucumbers with some fresh basil, bell peppers and slices of tomato, then add a slice of cheese and top with another piece of cucumber.
7. Use a toothpick to spear the stacks, then put back into the oven and bake until the cheese is completely melted and lightly browned i.e for about 10-15 minutes.
8. Remove from the oven and set aside to cool for a bit, serve and enjoy!

Chapter Twelve: Desserts

Everyone deserves some good dessert. I'd say it needs to be made a basic human right, who's with me?! I mean, who doesn't look forward to some dessert after a good meal? It doesn't matter if you have IBS, after eating a very tasty Low-FODMAP meal, leave some room for some Low-FODMAP dessert because the party's just getting started!

Low-Fodmap Brownies

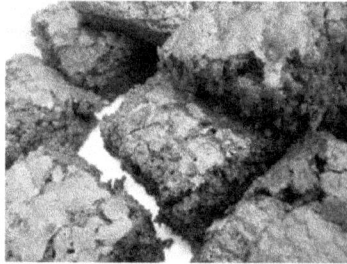

- Prep Time: 10 Minutes
- Cook Time: 30 minutes
- Yield: 13 servings
- Calories: 192 calories
- Nutrition Fact: **Sugars;** 9g **Proteins;** 10g **Fats;** 20g **Carbs;** 15g

What You'll Need

- Half a cup of brown sugar
- One(1) cup of Low-FODMAP chocolate chips
- One(1) cup of unsalted butter
- Half a cup of dark chocolate (roughly chopped)
- One(1) cup of granulated sugar
- One(1) cup of unsweetened cocoa powder
- Three(3) large eggs (at room temperature)
- Two(2) teaspoons of pure vanilla extract

- One(1) cup of gluten-free all purpose flour
- One(1) teaspoon of salt

Instructions

1. Preheat your oven to 350F.
2. Line a baking sheet with pieces of parchment paper.
3. Put half the amount of chopped chocolate and butter into a microwave safe bowl, put into the microwave and allow to melt, stirring at 30 seconds interval, until the mixture is completely smooth.
4. Remove from the microwave, then whisk in eggs, sugar and vanilla.
5. Add the flour, cocoa powder, salt, chocolate chunks and the other half of the chopped chocolates.
6. Use a rubber spatula to carefully fold the ingredients together, then pour batter into your pre-lined baking pan.
7. Put into the oven and bake for 30 minutes or until it passes the toothpick test, if it doesn't, bake for 5-7 minutes.
8. Remove from the oven and set on a cooling rack. Once cool, cut into pieces and serve.

Low-Fodmap Lemon Bar

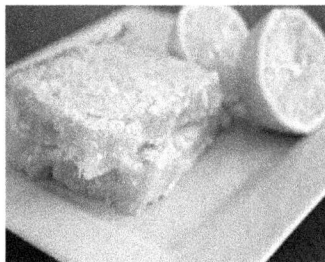

- Prep Time: 10 Minutes
- Cook Time: 50 minutes
- Yield: 16 servings
- Calories: 206 calories

- Nutrition Fact: **Sugars; 5g Proteins; 9g Fats; 15g Carbs; 10g**

What You'll Need

For the crust;

- Half a cup of unsalted butter (cut into pieces)
- Half a cup of white sugar
- One(1) cup of gluten free all purpose flour
- Two(2) tablespoons of water

For topping;

- A quarter cup of gluten-free all purpose flour
- Four(4) large eggs (lightly beaten)
- Powdered sugar (for dusting)
- One(1) cup of white sugar
- Four(4) tablespoons of freshly squeezed lemon juice

Instructions

1. Preheat your oven to 350F.
2. Coat or grease a baking pan and set aside.
3. Put the sugar and flour into a large mixing bowl, add the butter and mix by hand until crumbly, then pour in the water and mix until well combined.
4. Pour batter into greased pan and use the back of a spoon or spatula to flatten and level it.
5. Put into the oven and allow to bake for 25 minutes.
6. Put the eggs into a medium sized bowl, add the lemon juice, flour and sugar, stirring until smooth, then pour over baked crust.
7. Put back into the oven and bake for 25 minutes, then remove from oven and set on a cooling rack.
8. Sprinkle a thin layer of powdered sugar over it and cut into slices.
9. Serve.

Low-Fodmap Butterscotch

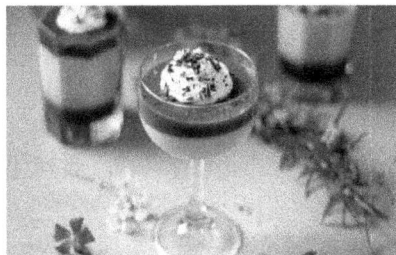

- Prep Time: 10 Minutes
- Cook Time: 15 Minutes
- Yield: 13 servings
- Calories: 263 calories
- Nutrition Fact: **Sugars;** 6.6g **Proteins;** 12g **Fats;** 16g **Carbs;** 8.4g

What You'll Need

- One(1) teaspoon of rum or scotch
- Three(3) egg yolks
- 40 grams of unsalted butter (at room temperature)
- One(1) teaspoon of vanilla extract
- One(1) cup of lactose-free whipping cream
- Three(3) tablespoons of water
- Two(2) tablespoons of cornstarch
- One(1) cup of lactose-free full fat milk
- One(1) cup of dark brown sugar
- Half a teaspoon of salt

Instructions

1. Pour the milk into a medium sized bowl, add the whipping cream and whisk until foamy.
2. Put the eggs and cornstarch into another bowl and whisk until well combined.

3. Pour the water into a medium-sized saucepan, set over medium heat, then add the sugar and salt, then cook for 5 minutes without stirring.
4. Slowly add the whipped cream mixture, whisking lightly until well incorporated, then bring to a boil.
5. Once boiled, remove half a cup of the mixture and pour into a separate bowl, then slowly add the egg yolks (to the bowl), stirring continuously so they don't scramble, then slowly pour the mixture into the saucepan, whisking lightly.
6. Set the heat on low and cook for 2 minutes or until the mixture thickens, then remove from heat.
7. Stir in vanilla, butter and scotch.
8. Allow to cool for a few minutes before serving into glasses.
9. Refrigerate overnight or for a couple of hours until it thickens .
10. Serve with any topping of your choice.

Low-Fodmap Cookies

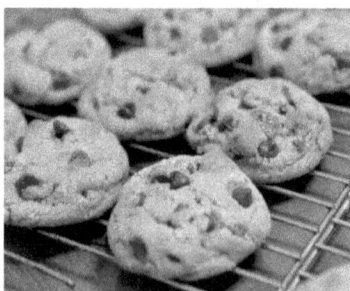

- Prep Time: 10 Minutes
- Cook Time: 10 Minutes
- Yield: 7 Servings
- Calories: calories
- Nutrition Fact: **Sugars;** 10g **Proteins;** 8g **Fats;** 13g **Carbs;** 28g

What You'll Need

- One(1) cup of brown sugar
- A quarter teaspoon of salt
- One(1) large egg
- One(1) teaspoon of pure vanilla extract
- One(1) cup of natural peanut butter
- Half a cup of dark chocolate chips

Instructions

1. Preheat your oven to 350F.
2. Throw all the ingredients into a large mixing bowl and stir using a wooden spoon or ladle until well combined.
3. Line a baking sheet with pieces of parchment.
4. Cut out a tablespoon of dough and roll it into a ball, then place it on the parchment lined baking sheet and press it flat with the broad side of the spoon.
5. Repeat the process in 4 above with the rest of the dough, and put the baking sheet into the oven
6. Bake for 10 minutes or until the edges have started to brown, then remove from the oven and let cool on the pan for a couple of minutes.

NOTE: The cookies will harden as they cool, so do not be bothered by how soft they are when removed from the oven.

Low-Fodmap Cupcake

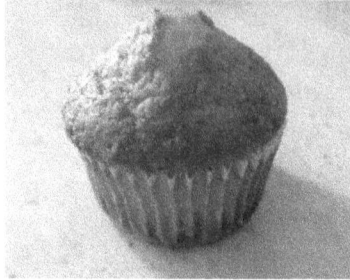

- Prep Time: 10 Minutes
- Cook Time: 35 Minutes
- Yield: 12 servings
- Calories: 197 calories
- Nutrition Fact: **Sugars;** 16g **Proteins;** 3g **Fats;** 6g **Carbs;** 33g

What You'll Need

- A quarter teaspoon of nutmeg
- One(1) cup of gluten-free all purpose flour
- Two(2) teaspoons of baking powder
- Half a teaspoon of cinnamon
- Two(2) tablespoons of milled linseed mixed with six(6) tablespoons of water
- Two(2) tablespoons of ground ginger
- A quarter cup of cold pressed rapeseed oil
- Half a cup of plant-based milk
- One (1) cup of sugar

Instructions

1. Preheat your oven to 350F.
2. Line a few cupcake tins with pieces of parchment paper.
3. Pour all your ingredients into a blender and pulse until smooth.
4. Then pour batter into tins and put them into the oven.

5. Bake for 35 minutes or until it passes the toothpick test, then remove from the oven and set to cool on a cooling rack.

Low-Fodmap Chocolate-Raspberry Pudding

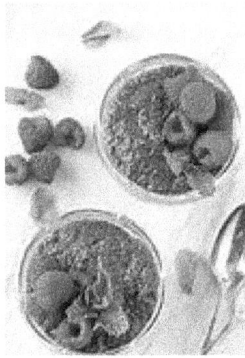

- Prep Time: 10 Minutes
- Cook Time: 0 Minutes
- Yield: 13 servings
- Calories: 192 calories
- Nutrition Fact: **Sugars;** 5g **Proteins;** 12g **Fats;** 17g **Carbs;** 14g

What You'll Need

- Half a cup of fresh raspberries
- Four(4) tablespoons of chia seeds
- Half a quarter teaspoon of raspberry extract
- Half a cup of unsweetened almond milk
- Two(2) tablespoons of pure maple syrup
- A pinch of salt
- One(1) tablespoon of unsweetened cocoa powder

Instructions

1. Put the maple syrup, chia seeds, raspberry extract, salt and cocoa powder into a glass jar with a lid.
2. Stir well into all the ingredients are combined, then slowly stir in the milk,

3. Cover the jar with the lid and refrigerate overnight or for 4-5 hours.
4. Once the pudding is set, transfer to serving dishes and serve topped with raspberries.

Low-Fodmap Flourless Cake

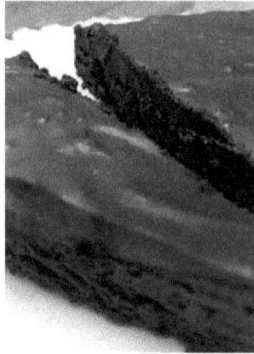

- Prep Time: 15 Minutes
- Cook Time: 30 Minutes
- Yield: 10 servings
- Calories: 192 calories
- Nutrition Fact: **Sugars;** 6g **Proteins;** 23g **Fats;** 19g **Carbs;** 18g

What You'll Need

- Half a cup of unsweetened cocoa powder (sifted)
- One(1) cup of white sugar
- Eight(8) tablespoons of unsalted butter
- Three(3) whole eggs
- Two (2) egg whites
- 170 grams of dark chocolate (chopped)

Instructions

1. Preheat your oven to 350F
2. Grease a baking dish, then line it with some pieces of parchment paper, then grease the parchment paper too.

3. Melt the butter and chocolate in a double boiler, then set aside once sufficiently melted.
4. Use an electric whisk to beat the egg whites until they form soft white peaks, then slowly add the sugar and beat again until well combined.
5. Pour the cocoa powder into a mixing bowl, then crack in the three whole eggs, mix until well combined.
6. Add the melted butter mixture and stir until well combined, then slowly fold in the egg white mixture and stir for 1-2 minutes until well mixed.
7. Pour batter into the baking pan and bake for 30 minutes.
8. Remove from the oven and set aside to cool for a few minutes. Let the cake cool completely before you remove it from the pan.
9. Cut and serve.

Chapter Thirteen: Homemade Cookies And Bars

Have you ever heard that the best cookies are made at home? You doubt? Well, I am going to be sharing some mouth-watering cookie recipes with you, how about you try them? If you are able to stop at one bite, you win, but if you take more than one, I win. So, what's it gonna be? Are you willing to get into this absolutely tasty challenge? Ok, let's start!

Low-Fodmap No-Bake Cookies

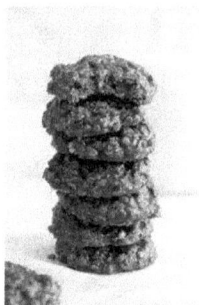

- Prep Time: 5 Minutes
- Cook Time: 5 minutes
- Yield: 20 servings
- Calories: 175 calories
- Nutrition Fact: **Sugars;** 4g **Proteins;** 16g **Fats;** 15g **Carbs;** 7g

What You'll Need

- A pinch of salt
- Two(2) cups of sugar
- A quarter cup of unsweetened cocoa powder
- Half a cup of butter
- One(1) cup of natural peanut butter

- Half a cup of unsweetened almond milk
- Three(3) cups of rolled oats
- One(1) teaspoon of pure vanilla extract

Instructions

1. Line a baking sheet or cookie tray with parchment paper.
2. Put the cocoa powder, milk, sugar and butter into a medium-sized saucepan, set over medium heat and bring to a boil, then remove from heat.
3. Add peanut butter, salt, oats and vanilla extract, stir, then scoop spoonfuls of the mixture onto parchment lined baking sheet.
4. Allow to cool for 30-45 minutes or until they harden completely.
5. Store in an airtight cookie jar and refrigerate and eat at leisure.

Low-Fodmap Raspberry Crumble Bars

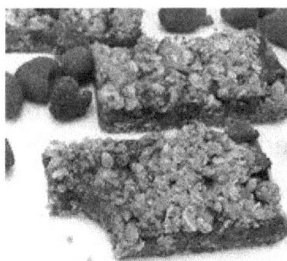

- Prep Time: 15 Minutes
- Cook Time: 40 Minutes
- Yield: 15 servings
- Calories: 218 Calories
- Nutrition Fact: **Sugars;** 2g **Proteins;** 9g **Fats;** 11g **Carbs;** 17.5g

What You'll Need

- One(1) cup of melted non-dairy butter
- Two(2) cups of raspberries
- One(1) cup of gluten-free oats
- Half a teaspoon of cinnamon
- Half a teaspoon of sea salt
- One(1) tablespoon of freshly squeezed lemon juice
- One(1) cup of brown sugar
- Two(2) teaspoons of cornstarch
- Two(2) tablespoons of maple syrup
- One(1) cup of gluten-free all purpose flour
- One (1) teaspoon of baking powder

Instructions

1. Put the lemon juice and raspberries into a small saucepan and set over medium heat.
2. Cook until the raspberries start to wilt, stirring occasionally to prevent the mixture from sticking to the bottom of the pot.
3. Add the cornstarch and maple syrup, stir and allow to cook for 5 more minutes.
4. Preheat your oven to 350F.
5. Put the flour, oats, cinnamon, salt and sugar into a large mixing bowl, mix to combine and stir in the melted butter. Stir until well combined.
6. Press half of the dough into the bottom of a parchment lined baking pan, then spoon the raspberry mixture over the dough.
7. Sprinkle the rest of the dough over the raspberry mixture, then place the pan into the oven and allow to bake for 40 minutes.
8. Remove from the oven and allow to cool for 5-10 minutes, then cut into slices and serve or store in an airtight container for up to 5 days.

Low-Fodmap Peanut Butter Cookies

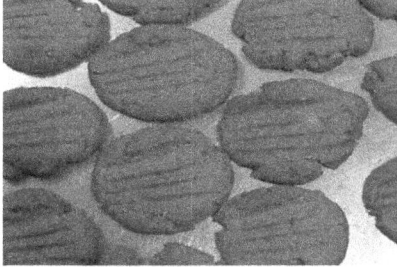

- Prep Time: Minutes
- Cook Time: 12 Minutes
- Yield: 14 Servings
- Calories: 193 Calories
- Nutrition Fact: **Sugars;** 4g **Proteins;** 9g **Fats;** 18g **Carbs;** 12g

What You'll Need

- One(1) large egg
- One(1) teaspoon of baking soda
- One(1) cup of gluten-free all purpose flour
- Eight(8) tablespoons of unsalted butter
- A cup of gluten free oats
- A quarter teaspoon of salt
- One(1) teaspoon of pure vanilla extract
- A cup of sugar
- One(1) teaspoon of baking soda
- Half a cup of peanut butter

Instructions

1. Preheat your oven to 350F.
2. Line a cookie sheet with pieces of parchment paper.

3. Put the baking soda, gluten-free flour and salt into a small bowl and mix until well combined, then set aside.
4. Put the peanut butter, sugar, butter and vanilla extract into a bowl and beat with an electric mixer for three minutes on high.
5. Crack in the egg and continue to beat, then slowly fold in the dry ingredients from the set aside bowl, then stir to combine.
6. Slowly stir in the oats and mix until well combined.
7. Use an ice cream or cookie scoop to scoop the dough onto the baking sheet and bake for 12 minutes.
8. Remove from oven and set on a cooling rack and allow to cool for a few minutes.
9. Serve and enjoy!

Low-Fodmap Oatmeal Chip Bars

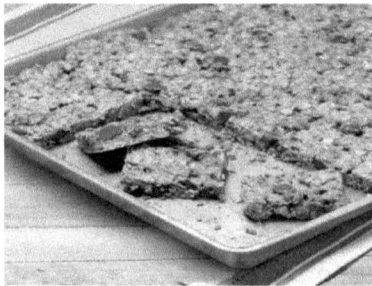

- Prep Time: 20 Minutes
- Cook Time: 20 Minutes
- Yield: 12 Servings
- Calories: 179 Calories
- Nutrition Fact: **Sugars;** 7g **Proteins;** 5g **Fats;** 8g **Carbs;** 23g

What You'll Need

- Six(6) cups of gluten-free oats
- Four(4) large eggs

- One(1) cup of gluten-free butterscotch chips
- Half a cup of brown sugar
- One(1) cup of semi-sweet chocolate chips
- One(1) cup of ripe bananas (mashed)
- One(1) cup of peanut butter
- Half a teaspoon of salt

Instructions

1. Put the eggs and brown sugar into a large bowl and beat until well blended.
2. Add the peanut butter, bananas and salt and stir until well combined.
3. Stir in the butterscotch, oats and chocolate chips and mix until well incorporated.
4. Preheat your oven to 350F.
5. Coat a baking pan with cooking spray and pour batter into it.
6. Bake for 25 minutes, remove from oven and allow to cool before cutting into bars.

Low-Fodmap Cookie Dough Balls

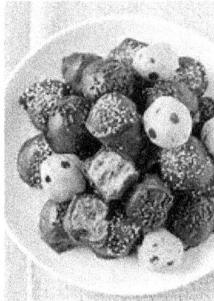

- Prep Time: 15 Minutes
- Cook Time: 0 Minutes
- Yield: 16 Servings
- Calories: 241 Calories
- Nutrition Fact: **Sugars;** 7g **Proteins;** 13g **Fats;** 15g **Carbs;** 21g

What You'll Need

- One(1) cup of gluten-free all purpose flour
- Half a cup of unsalted butter (softened)
- A quarter teaspoon of salt
- Half a cup of dairy-free chocolate chips
- A quarter cup of granulated sugar
- Two(2) teaspoons of neutral oil
- Half a cup of dark brown sugar
- One(1) teaspoon of pure vanilla extract

Instructions

1. Put the butter and sugar into a bowl and beat until smooth and fluffy.
2. Stir in the salt and vanilla, then add the flour and stir until well combined.
3. Add half of the chocolate chips and stir lightly (careful not to mash the chocolate chips).
4. Mold the dough into small round balls and place on the lined baking sheet.
5. Refrigerate for about thirty minutes or until firm.
6. Put the rest of the chocolate chips into a microwave friendly bowl, put it into the microwave and allow to melt, stirring at 15 seconds interval.
7. Remove from microwave and add the oil, stir until well combined, then dip each dough ball into the chocolate until completely coated, then place back into the lined baking sheet.
8. Decorate to your preference, then put the dough in the fridge until the chocolate hardens, then serve!

Chapter Fourteen: Meal Prep

If you find it hard to keep to time and always find yourself scrambling to make something to take to work, then you've probably never heard of meal prep. Yes! It saves time, it saves you the stress and it always turns out yummy! Don't know what meal prepping is? Well, it is just making meals, in this case Low-FODMAP meals ahead of time. So you have already made meals, any time you want! For breakfast, lunch or dinner!

Low-Fodmap Chickpea Salad

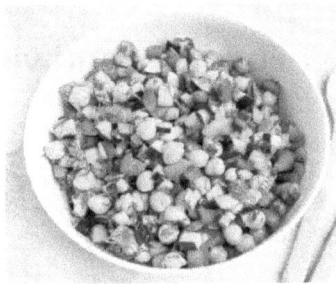

- Prep Time: 10 Minutes
- Cook Time: 0 Minutes
- Yield: 8 Servings
- Calories: 225 Calories
- Nutrition Fact: **Sugars;** 4g **Proteins;** 20g **Fats;** 12g **Carbs;** 5g

What You'll Need

- Half a piece of green pepper (diced)
- One(1) teaspoon of fresh scallions (green part only)
- One(1) red bell pepper (chopped)
- One(1) medium sized cucumber (chopped)
- One(1) cup of fresh parsley
- A can of chickpeas (drained and rinsed)

For the dressing;

- Two(2) tablespoons of freshly squeezed lemon juice
- Three(3) tablespoons of olive oil
- Two(2) tablespoons of maple syrup
- Two(2) tablespoons of red wine vinegar

Instructions

1. Pour all the dressing ingredients into a medium sized mixing bowl, whisk until well combined.
2. Put all the other ingredients into a large bowl, then pour the dressing over it and toss until fully coated, then Sha the salad into airtight containers and refrigerate for up to four days.
3. Alternatively, you could keep the dressing in a lidded glass jar and store the salad in small airtight containers and pour some dressing in them only when you are ready to eat.

Low-Fodmap Sandwich

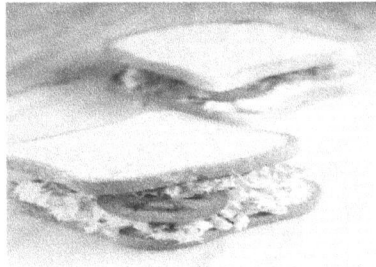

- Prep Time: 10 Minutes
- Cook Time: 0 Minutes
- Yield: 6 Servings
- Calories: 156 Calories
- Nutrition Fact: **Sugars;** 1g **Proteins;** 15 **Fats;** 11g **Carbs;** 18g

What You'll Need

- Slices of Low-FODMAP bread
- One(1) can of tuna
- One(1) tablespoon of minced chives

124

- Four tomatoes (sliced)
- Five(5) romaine lettuce leaves
- Two(1) tablespoons of mayonnaise
- A quarter cup of diced Cucumber
- Two(2) teaspoons of mustard
- Two(2) tablespoons of Kalamata olives

Instructions

1. Put the tuna, chives, mustard, mayonnaise and cucumber into a medium sized bowl, stir until well combined, then transfer into airtight containers and refrigerate for up to five days.
2. When ready to eat, spread some of the tuna mixture onto two slices of Low-FODMAP bread, then top with lettuce and tomato slices.
3. If you want some crust to your sandwich, you can toast your bread, or grill the sandwich a bit on a skillet over medium heat.

Low-Fodmap Rice Bowl

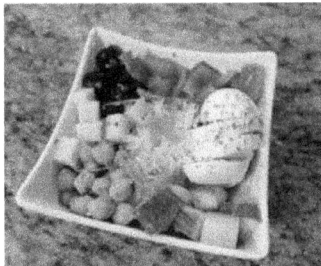

- Prep Time: 15 Minutes
- Cook Time: 0 Minutes
- Yield: 4 Servings
- Calories: 300 Calories

- Nutrition Fact: **Sugars;** 1g **Proteins;** 16g **Fats;** 13g **Carbs;** 6g

What You'll Need

- One(1) cup of canned chickpeas (rinsed and drained)
- A quarter cup of olive oil
- One(1) cucumber (chopped)
- A quarter cup of fresh mint (chopped)
- A quarter cup of balsamic vinegar
- Three(3) cups of cooked quinoa
- 150 grams of crumbled feta cheese
- Half a cup of cherry tomatoes (halved)
- Four(4) spring onions (green part only)
- Four(4) boiled eggs
- One(1) red pepper (diced)
- One(1) cup of Kalamata olives

Instructions

1. Put the vinegar and olive oil into a bowl, stir until combined, then pour into an airtight jar and refrigerate for up to 4 days.
2. Share the rest of the ingredients in meal prep containers and refrigerate for up to 4 days too.
3. Serve with a light drizzle of dressing. Enjoy at anytime of the day!

Low-Fodmap Sausages

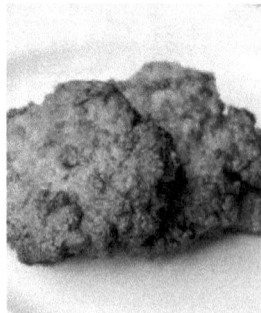

- Prep Time: 10 Minutes
- Cook Time: 15 Minutes
- Yield: 14 Servings
- Calories: 174 Calories
- Nutrition Fact: **Sugars;** 1g **Proteins;** 6.2g **Fats;** 13.8 **Carbs;** 3g

What You'll Need

- One(1) tablespoon of pure maple syrup
- Two(2) tablespoons of ground pork
- One (1) teaspoon of ground pepper
- One(1) teaspoon of salt
- Four(4) teaspoons of ground sage
- Half a teaspoon of crushed red pepper flakes

Instructions

1. Put all the ingredients into a bowl, mix by hand and cut out small amounts of it and form small patties.
2. Coat a small skillet with cooking spray and place the patties on it and cook on each side until brown.
3. Put into airtight containers and refrigerate.
4. Microwave when you are ready to eat and serve with some Low-FODMAP bread.

Low-Fodmap Spanish Rice

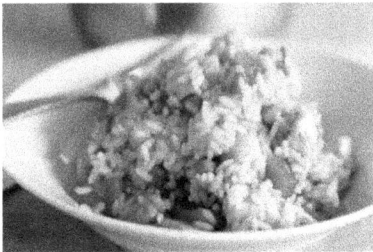

- Prep Time: 10 Minutes
- Cook Time: 15 Minutes
- Yield: 2 Servings

- Calories: 264 Calories
- Nutrition Fact: **Sugars;** 0.6g **Proteins;** 8.5g **Fats;** 6.5g **Carbs;** 19g

What You'll Need

- Half a piece of red pepper
- Three(3) Finely sliced spring onions (green part only)
- One(1) teaspoon of oregano
- 200 grams of rice
- One(1) teaspoon of cumin
- Three(3) tablespoons of peas
- One(1) teaspoon of turmeric
- Half a teaspoon of chilli Pepper
- Two(2) tablespoons of olive oil
- One(1) teaspoon of asafoetida
- Roasted or cooked chicken
- 250ml of water

Instructions

1. Put the oil into a medium sized frying pan, allow to simmer for a few seconds, then add the spring onions, stir fry for five minutes.
2. Add the chili, rice, oregano, turmeric, asafoetida and cumin, then pour in water and bring to a boil.
3. Stir and cook on low for 15 minutes.
4. Add a little more water once the rice dried out.
5. Dice the red pepper and throw it into the mix, stir and add the peas and chicken.
6. Then cook for five more minutes.
7. Once the rice is ready, allow to cool for 10 minutes, then serve into meal prep bowls, then refrigerate
8. When you are ready to eat, just microwave and serve!

Chapter Fifteen: Low-Fodmap Juices

Time to quench your thirst... literally! It is such a chore going through the list of ingredients on every store bought pack of juice or beverage. But what can you do? Is there a better choice? Well, yeah. You can go natural! Yes, you can make those tasty juices you crave without worrying about the FODMAP content. No jokes! The recipes below are Low-FODMAP and absolutely tasty!

Low-Fodmap Green Smoothie

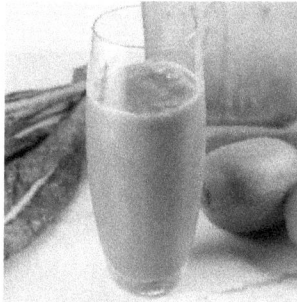

- Prep Time: 5 Minutes
- Cook Time: 0 Minutes
- Yield: 2 Servings
- Calories: 132 Calories
- Nutrition Fact: **Sugars;** 25g **Proteins;** 3g **Fats;** 1g **Carbs;** 33g

What You'll Need

- Two(2) cups of ice cubes
- A cup of seedless green grapes
- Two(2) cups of baby spinach
- One(1) kiwi (peeled and cut into chunks)
- One(1) big cucumber (cut into chunks)

- Two(2) tablespoons of water

Instructions

1. Put all the ingredients (except ice) into a blender, pulse on medium for 3-5 minutes, then increase the speed and blend until pureed and smooth.
2. Add about half the amount of ice and pulse again until frosty.
3. Add some more ice and pulse until the ice is broken into tiny little chunks, then serve immediately.
4. You could also do the recipe without ice and put in whole ice cubes when you are ready to drink. So it won't be frosty, but it will

Low-Fodmap Turmeric, Ginger Lemon Juice

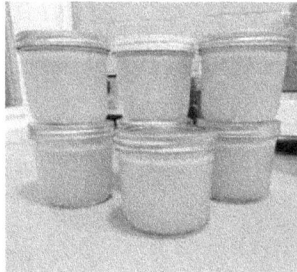

- Prep Time: 5 Minutes
- Cook Time: 0 Minutes
- Yield: 7 Servings
- Calories: 161 Calories
- Nutrition Fact: **Sugars;** 7g **Proteins;** 10g **Fats;** 7g **Carbs;** 2g

What You'll Need

- Four(4) cups of water
- Five lemons (peeled)
- 30 grams of fresh ginger (cut into pieces)
- A quarter cup of maple syrup

- 30 grams of fresh turmeric root (cut into pieces)

Instructions

1. Put the ingredients (except water and maple syrup) into a juicer. Preferably one at a time.
2. Once you have gotten the juice, pour it into a blender and add the rest of the ingredients, pulse on high for 30 seconds to a minute.
3. Serve over ice, or store in lidded jars for later.

Low-Fodmap Carrot Juice

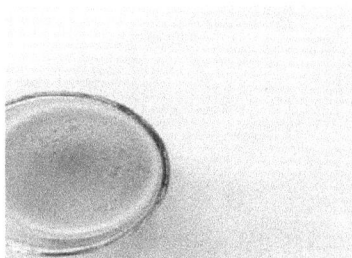

- Prep Time: 10 Minutes
- Cook Time: 5 Minutes
- Yield: 2 Servings
- Calories: 202 Calories
- Nutrition Fact: **Sugars;** 20g **Proteins;** 5g **Fats;** 1g **Carbs;** 47g

What You'll Need

- A small piece of ginger (peeled)
- One(1) tablespoon of bee pollen
- Ten(10) carrots (cut off the tops)
- Four(4) oranges (cut and peel)
- Ice cubes

Instructions

1. Run your carrots, oranges and ginger through a juicer.

2. Once they are all juiced, put them into a bowl and add the bee pollen, whisk until well combined.
3. Serve over ice.

Low-Fodmap Tomato Juice

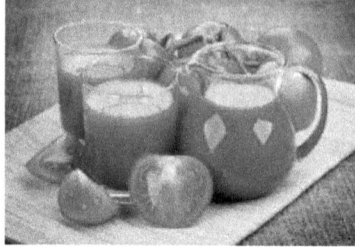

- Prep Time: 5 Minutes
- Cook Time: 0 Minutes
- Yield: 3 Servings
- Calories: 180 Calories
- Nutrition Fact: **Sugars;** 10g **Proteins;** 2g **Fats;** 0.6g **Carbs;** 11g

What You'll Need

- Five(5) grams of horseradish
- A dash of Tabasco
- 50ml of vodka (optional)
- A quarter cup of lemon juice
- One (1) cup of tomato juice
- Pepper and salt to taste
- A dash of Worcestershire sauce
- Half a tablespoon of dry Sherry
- Two(2) grams of celery seed

Instructions

1. Pour all ingredients into a blender (if it is not enough, do it in batches), set on high and pulse for 2-3 minutes.
2. Transfer to a pitcher and serve over ice.

Low-Fodmap Lemonade

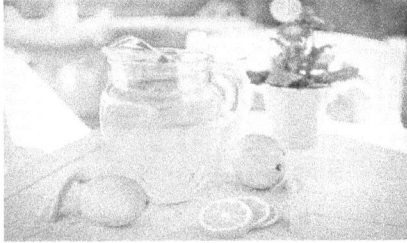

- Prep Time: 15 Minutes
- Cook Time: 0 Minutes
- Yield: 10 Servings
- Calories: 76 Calories
- Nutrition Fact: **Sugars;** 4g **Proteins;** 0.8g **Fats;** 0.2g **Carbs;** 2g

What You'll Need

- Eight(8) cups of water
- One(1) cup of sugar
- Two(2) cups of freshly squeezed lemon juice

Instructions

1. Pour a cup of water into a sauce pan, add the sugar and set over medium heat and allow to boil.
2. Remove from heat and allow to cool for about 30 minutes.
3. Once cooled, pour into a pitcher, add the rest of the water, and lemon juice.
4. Stir and serve over ice, or refrigerate until ready to consume.

Low-Fodmap Strawberry Juice

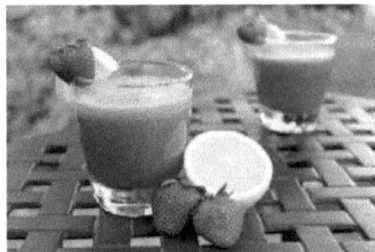

- Prep Time: 10 Minutes
- Cook Time: 0 Minutes
- Yield: 4 Servings
- Calories: Calories
- Nutrition Fact: **Sugars;** 5g **Proteins;** 1.3g **Fats;** 0.7g **Carbs;** 3g

What You'll Need

- A cup of ice
- A couple of lemon slices (to garnish)
- Three cups of natural lemon tea
- Two(2) tablespoons of sugar
- Two(2) tablespoons of freshly squeezed lemon juice
- One(1) cup of frozen strawberries

Instructions

1. To brew your tea, put the teabags into a lidded jar and soak overnight.
2. Put the strawberries, brewed tea, sugar and lemon juice into a blender, pulse on high for 2-3 minutes or until smooth, then add ice and pulse until frosty.
3. Serve garnished with lemon slices. Enjoy!

Conclusion

Dealing with IBS is not easy, it's uncomfortable and sometimes painful, but the low-FODMAP diet has come to change all that. It has become that little speck of light in a cave of utter darkness, but it can't work on its own. You have a huge role to play also, you have to follow your dieticians suggestions to the letter. If you slack, you alone will suffer, so have some fun learning how to make these beginner-friendly recipes, and before you know it, you'll feel absolutely amazing and it would be time to get off the diet. Just like that! It's a win-win situation. So live, eat and enjoy!

Part 2

Introduction

Health concerns in recent decades have grown in step with population growth. Fortunately, this has also been accompanied by an explosion in research and medical breakthroughs. Institutional agencies and individual researchers have regularly come out with findings and remedies that are now benefiting many people health-wise. One of the major fields in health research where advances regularly make the headlines is in diet or the food people eat. Partly, it is a recognition of the overriding importance of one part of our body in preventing illnesses and maintaining over-all health: our gut. If you are one of those people who are afflicted with irritable bowel syndrome or any other related disorder, this book will help you tremendously.

Thanks again for downloading this book, I hope you enjoy it!

Chapter 1: Common Gut Problems

You do your best to remain healthy and you follow the usual recommendations to stay in tip-top shape. You exercise regularly, get enough sleep, have periodic checkups, take vitamins and minerals, and eat right—or so you thought. But still something is wrong with your body and you discover later that poor gut health is the unexpected culprit. It is sabotaging all the hard work and supplementation. Many health experts consider the digestive system as the foundation of our wellbeing, and for good reason. It impacts so many body processes. If it is in good condition, you can perform at the optimum level whether at work or at the gym.

Poor gut health can actually cause your body many problems. It can impair the immune system, making you more susceptible to diseases. It can also cause hormonal imbalance throughout your body. What causes this is the vast quantity of neurons in your stomach that discharge the same neurotransmitters found in the brain. So when your gastrointestinal tract equilibrium is upset, your body and mood are also thrown into chaos. This happens because the digestive system is one major roadway from the mouth to the anus. When it becomes leaky or more permeable, it can cause damage to the gastrointestinal tract.

One of the many factors that can make the gut leaky is poor food choices. Poor gut health is also known to lead to other seemingly unrelated conditions like allergies, inflammations, skin conditions, impaired performance, and even unwanted weight gain.

One of the major usual consequences of such a condition is irritable bowel syndrome (IBS). IBS is a common malady that affects the colon or large intestine. It is a chronic condition that causes constipation, abdominal pain, cramping, gas, diarrhea, and bloating. Also, IBS needs long-term management instead of one-time only treatment.

Some people with IBS can have severe signs and symptoms but other afflicted people can control it by managing diet along with other measures. Symptoms vary from person to person with some people needing counseling and others, medication. For most patients, IBS is a persistent, long-term condition that alternately gets worse and better. It tends to recur in periods lasting from a few days to a few months usually after one has eaten certain foods or during stressful situations. It is estimated to affect 20% of the population—a huge number. And the ailment is usually life-long.

IBS has no cure, but it can be managed through appropriate dietary adjustments and lifestyle changes. Thus, it is important to identify the foods that can trigger it, exercise regularly, and minimize exposure to stressful situations.

Because of the lack of cure and the resultant painful and debilitating condition, IBS can also cause people anxiety and depression. It negatively affects your over-all quality of life and emotional state. Restoring your wellbeing would require no less than healing your gut lining. A primary step towards this objective is removing the stress-causing food and toxins from your diet.

Bloating is another major discomfort that afflicts our gut. This condition is not confined to holiday binge eating. An estimated 10% of Americans suffer from this disorder on a regular basis. In more severe cases, it can cause abdominal swelling.

Like IBS, bloating and gas are generally connected to the type of food you eat, so making changes in diet can do wonders. Gas in the abdomen is the next major cause of bloating. Half of this gas is produced by food-digesting bacteria in the gut. If the gastrointestinal tract is malfunctioning and cannot move the gas efficiently, bloating and discomfort ensue. Experts identify certain types of food, sweeteners, and dairy products that can cause gassiness, bloating, and other intestinal distress and therefore must be avoided.

Correct knowledge is crucial in the proper application of the FODMAP concept. For instance, whole grains which are noted for their many health benefits and can at times trigger bloating and gas disorder. Yet what makes grains very healthy is their high fiber content. Still one problem with fiber is that it is an indigestible carbohydrate. So the right thing to do is to gradually, not abruptly, increase the amount of fiber in your diet as it can cause gas, bloating, and constipation.

Slowly increasing the fiber in your diet will allow your body enough time to adjust. Joanne L. Slavin, PhD, RD, professor of food science and nutrition at the University of Minnesota, recommends drinking plenty of water while eating high-fiber foods. Fiber is able to move through the digestive system and prevents bloating and constipation, especially when one is drinking enough liquids regularly. This is because fiber absorbs water well.

Fortunately, two Australian researchers, Sue Shepherd and Peter Gibson, were able to isolate and identify the main ingredients that cause IBS and other digestive woes as well as the foods that usually contain these ingredients. Out of the names of those small chain sugars and fibers, they coined the now famous acronym FODMAP.

Chapter 2: How The Fodmap Concept Helps

What are FODMAPs?

FODMAP sounds like a strange military term or an intelligence-gathering activity using satellites. In reality, it stands for a number of carbohydrates that your body finds hard to digest properly.
FODMAP stands for:

Fermentable

Oligosaccharides (Fructans and Galacto-oligosaccharides – GOS)
Disaccharides (Lactose, milk sugar)
Monosaccharides (excess fructose)

And

Polyols (sugar alcohols such as mannitol and sorbitol)
In other words, FODMAP means Fermentable Oligosaccharides, Disaccharides, Monosaccharides, And Polyols. These are all types of carbohydrates found in many fruits, vegetables, and grains. Examples of foods high in FODMAPs are:
1. **Lactols** – Milk, Custard, Ice Cream, Yogurt, Milk powder, Ricotta cheese, Cottage cheese

2. **Excess fructose** – Apples, Boysenberry, Figs, Mango, Pears, Watermelon, Asparagus, Artichoke, Sugar, Snap peas, High Fructose corn syrup, Honey, Agave

3. **Fructans** - Dried fruit, Nectarine, Persimmon, Watermelon, Artichoke, Garlic, Onion, Wheat, Barley, Rye, Chicory rooty extract, Inulin additives

4. **GOS** – Legumes, Pistachios, Cashews

5. **Polyols** – Apples, Apricots, Nectarine, Blackberries, Peach, Pears, Cauliflowers, Mushrooms, Sugar, Alcohol, Additives: isomalt, mannitol, sorbitol, maltitol

In essence, FODMAPs consist of certain small chain carbohydrates (sugars and fibers) that your small intestine often has difficult absorbing. FODMAPs are present in large quantities in diets and commonly found in daily foods and some medicines. It is estimated that up to 75% of those afflicted by IBS will directly benefit from the removal of FODMAPs from their diets. Similarly, studies reveal that a low FODMAP diet alleviates IBS-related gastrointestinal (GI) symptoms like gas, bloating, pain, and change in bowel habits.

How do FODMAPs cause the symptoms for individuals with IBS? It stems principally from the very small carbohydrate structure of FODMAPs. With such a configuration, they can draw water into the small intestine. This action causes diarrhea in a person with an intestine that is moving fast. If you are often afflicted with constipation, it feels like you are carrying a balloon filled with water inside your gut. In addition, another problem happens as the microbes in your intestine try to digest the FODMAPs that you ingested. The microbes end up fermenting the hard-to-digest FODMAPs thus producing gas. This gas stretches the intestine, causing bloating, abdominal pain, and cramping in vulnerable individuals. When gas and water come together in the intestine, it can promote constipation and diarrhea owing to the changes in the movement of the intestine. Statistics show that almost 20% of women often suffer from chronic constipation while 14% are regularly afflicted by pain or bloating. It used to be that the usual suspect was gluten which ballooned into a full-blown food craze. Everything changed after the scientists who originally blamed gluten conducted a study of the substance in comparison with FODMAPs. They found that only 8% of the subjects experienced worse symptoms through gluten while the 92% got it through FODMAPs. So FODMAPS, they realized, are the real troublemaker. Dr. Jessica

Biesiekierski, one of the world's leading gluten experts, stated that those who believe they have gluten sensitivity would benefit from eating fewer FODMAPs.

TIP: Always consult a doctor if you feel you have GI symptoms. Never perform a self-diagnosis. It is because there is a possibility that those symptoms are signs of far more serious ailments like colon cancer and celiac diseases, or inflammatory bowel disease. Likewise, ovarian cancer may be the real culprit for your bloating and other changes in bowel habits. Only a licensed medical professional can properly identify your actual illness.

How the FODMAP concept can really help

To better understand how FODMAPs come into the picture in the fight to maintain a healthy gut, it would be crucial to first understand more what happens inside your digestive system.

First, a perfect ecosystem supposedly exists in your gut where your body digests food. Involved in that activity inside you are trillions of bacteria that help digest what you eat and fight infections. The more diverse that microbial community, the healthier you will be. Unfortunately, that ecosystem can easily be disrupted by many new things like artificial sweeteners and alcoholism which can put your health into a tailspin.

This is where the concept of FODMAPs becomes highly relevant. FODMAPs are molecules in the following types of sugar: fructose, fructans, lactose, galactans, and polyols. Being osmotic, they pull water during digestion into the small intestine. That process can also cause bloating, diarrhea, and abdominal pain. And as these foods are broken down by bacteria in the large intestine, they undergo fermentation that produces gas and causes discomforts. The problem is most severe in people who cannot tolerate even small amounts of FODMAPs. The remedy that experts realized is to temporarily restrict FODMAPs from entering the body. As a result, diets low in FODMAPs were developed.

Studies show that these food formulations were more effective in alleviating the suffering of afflicted people than medications and similar interventions. Symptoms like bloating and pain were effectively relieved in at least 75% of the cases. Dr. Mullin, one of the researchers, even noted weight loss as one of the effects on his patients as balancing gut bacteria could lessen food cravings.

FODMAPs are difficult to digest and absorb and so they significantly correlate with the symptoms commonly seen in all types of gastrointestinal disorders. In one study, the symptoms were clearly controlled in a vast majority of the subjects after removing the FODMAPs from the diet. Those sugar molecules, of course, did not trigger the development of IBS.

This is how you do it. Remove foods high in FODMAPs from your diet for a period of two to six weeks until the symptoms disappear or are substantially lessened. This would also mean the temporary disappearance of most bread from your table due to the gluten factor. When the symptoms have been sufficiently dispelled, bring back the FODMAP gradually one food per group every three days into your diet. If the symptoms reappear, it could mean that you are intolerant to, say, lactose. Continue the experiment with the goal of determining the quantity of the trigger foods that you can comfortably handle.

Otherwise, if no symptoms return even after reintroducing everything in your diet, it could mean that a simple rebalancing in your gut bacteria is all that is needed. It is important to ultimately bring back only those high-FODMAP foods that are not only healthy but are also not among the triggers. Those kinds of food have other invaluable health contributions like minimizing the risk of obesity and cancer. Likewise, the fiber in fruits, beans, whole grains, and similar foods, although indigestible, provides a home for the good bacteria to ensure that your gut remains always healthy.

This kind of low-FODMAP diet is particularly beneficial for mothers who have just taken heavy dosages of antibiotics as a result of Caesarian operation, dental surgery, and similar procedures that end up wreaking havoc on their internal ecosystems. The low-FODMAP diet can also help anyone in achieving healthy weight loss. When you feel pleased with the result, you will be strongly motivated to keep eating right.

Chapter 3: Low-Fodmap Recipes

1. Beef Bourguignon

Ingredients:

- 500g/18-oz chuck steak
- ¼ cup tapioca flour
- 1 tsp dry rosemary
- 1 tsp cumin powder
- 2 carrots
- 2 cups dry red wine
- 1 bayleaf
- 1 tbsp tomato paste
- Salt & Pepper
- 2 zucchini

Instructions

1. Season flour to taste with cumin powder, pepper, and salt. Add the meat and have it well-coated in the mixture by stirring.
2. Fry meat in the frying pan using a little coconut oil until it is brown.
3. Bring out meat from pan. Pour ½ cup of wine into pan and heat it as you scrape residue.
4. Chop roughly peeled zucchini and carrots.
5. Combine all prepared ingredients in a casserole or slow cooker and stir to mix well.
6. For 5 hours, cook on auto in slow cooker; in casserole about 2 hours.

2. Salmon With Mustard, Dill, And Maple

Ingredients: Serves 2-3

- 1/4 tsp paprika
- 2 tbsp pure maple syrup
- 1 tbsp Dijon mustard
- 1-2 tbsp chopped fresh dill
- 6-8 oz salmon
- 1 lemon (1/2 of the lemon sliced and other half to squeeze over salmon)
- 1 tbsp sliced garlic scapes (can sub in spring onion greens)
- Salt and pepper, to taste

Instructions

1. Preheat oven to 450°F. Prepare a baking sheet with parchment paper.
2. Mix paprika, maple syrup, mustard, salt and pepper in small bowl.
3. On the baking sheet put the salmon.
4. Take the maple syrup, mustard, paprika mixture and spread evenly on the salmon
5. Put 4-5 slices of lemon over salmon, drizzle additional lemon juice on it.
6. Bake at least 15 minutes in oven or up to the point it is cooked thoroughly.
7. Take out salmon from oven and sprinkle fresh dill and garlic scapes on it.

3. Quick Lamb Tagine

Ingredients:
- A small pot of Greek yoghurt
- 500g/17.6-oz lamb neck fillets
- 4 spring onions (green tops only)
- 1 tsp garam masala
- 500g/17.6-oz mixed color tomatoes
- 1 tbsp sesame seeds
- 1 pinch saffron
- 1 tbsp cumin seeds
- ½ green capsicum
- Salt & pepper
- 1 fresh chilli
- 1 large aubergine
- 2 tbsp chopped coriander

Instructions

1. Microwave the aubergine for 7 minutes.
2. Chop into pieces the lamb and add garam masala, pepper, and salt.
3. Add in a frying pan 1 tablespoon of oil and when hot toss in the lamb.
4. Toast in a pan the cumin seeds and sesame seeds, then remove.
5. Slice aubergine in half. Put together with lamb in the pan with the cut side down.
6. Half fill a cup with boiled water and add into it the saffron.
7. Add 2 tbsp oil into another frying pan and heat. Cut and place into the pan spring onions, tomatoes, chili and green pepper.
8. Pour into pan water with saffron and boil in high heat.
9. Transfer into a platter and sprinkle with coriander and seeds.
10. Yogurt should be on platter's side.

4. Tzatziki Sauce-Flavored Juicy Turkey Burgers

Ingredients:

- ¼ cup diced cucumber
- 1 cup plain Greek yogurt (can substitute plain lactose free yogurt)
- 1 lb ground dark meat turkey
- 1 cup reduced-fat feta cheese
- Juice of ½ or 1 lemon
- ½ cup pitted Kalamata olives, halved

For the Tzatziki Sauce:

- ½ cup chopped fresh dill
- Juice of ¼ lemon
- 1 lb ground white meat turkey
- **2 tbsp chopped fresh dill**

Instructions

1. Mix well all ingredients together, and make 11 burgers. Grill until heat is 165°F. (keep frozen leftover patties for use later)
2. Making Tzatziki sauce: Mix in a small bowl all ingredients. You can use this delicious sauce to flavor your burger.

5. Baked Brie With Cranberry Chutney

Ingredients:

- 2 tsp dairy free butter
- 1 (8-oz) package brie cheese (with rind)
- 2 tbsp chopped pecans
- 2 tbsp packed brown sugar
- ¼ cranberry chutney

Instructions

1. Prepare oven by preheating to 350°F.
2. Lightly coat a small ovenproof dish with nonstick cooking spray.
3. In the small dish, put in the brie (you can cut top if you want)
4. Put chutney on top of brie like cake frosting.
5. Sprinkle pecans over chutney and brown sugar over pecans.
6. Using butter without dairy, dot the top.
7. For 15-18 minutes, bake until brie is very soft.
8. Bring heat to 425°F and bake for an additional 5 minutes.
9. Brie will be starting to melt on the bottom and the sugar will be bubbling on the top.
10. This dish goes well with rice cakes or gluten-free crackers.

6. Yummy Fish Tacos

Ingredients:

- 1 tsp lime juice
- 2 tacos per person
- 1 tbsp mayonnaise
- 3 ounces firm fleshed fish such as cod
- ½ cup lettuce leaves
- 1/8 tsp Chipotle chili powder
- 2 tsp grapeseed oil or other high smoking point cooking oil
- ¼ cup chopped tomatoes
- salt and pepper, to taste
- 1/8 avocado, sliced
- 1/8 tsp cumin
- 1 teaspoon lime zest
- 2 corn tortillas
- **¼ cup finely shredded cheddar and/or Monterey Jack cheese**

Instructions:

1. Flavor the fish with pepper, salt, chipotle chili powder, and cumin, then set aside.
2. Put 2 teaspoons of oil in a medium skillet and warm it to average heat.
3. Cook fish side down in skillet for 4 minutes then turn the other side and cook for 4 more minutes or until cooked thoroughly and flaking.
4. Prepare lime aioli as you cook the fish.
5. Mix lime juice, mayonnaise, salt, lime zest, and pepper to taste in a dish.
6. Microwave to warm tortillas or in another skillet in low heat.
7. Cut fish into small pieces when it is thoroughly cooked.
8. Flavor corn tortillas by layering these with avocado, lettuce, fish, tomato, and shredded cheese.
9. Sprinkle lime aioli on tortilla.

7. Buffalo Chicken Dip

Ingredients: Serves 12

- Blue corn chips
- 2 medium-sized boneless, skinless, chicken breast (approximately ½ pound)
- 1 cup each grated sharp cheddar and grated asiago
- 1 tbsp fresh chives, chopped
- ½ cup FODMAP Free Ranch Dressing
- ½ cup FODMAP Free Buffalo Wing Sauce
- 8 oz cream cheese, softened
- 2 scallions, diced (green part only)
- 1 tsp salt

Instructions:

1. Wash chicken using cold water.
2. Cut chicken breasts in half and place in medium size pan together with chopped chives and salt, then pour in water, to cover.
3. As it boils, decrease the heat and for 15-20 minutes allow to simmer while waiting for chicken to be thoroughly cooked.
4. Bring out chicken and let it cool slightly.
5. Pull chicken into shreds with your hands. For faster shredding, chicken can be chopped into chunks first.
6. Spread the cream cheese in a 1-quart shallow baking dish. Dish should be ungreased.
7. Over the cheese, spread the shredded chicken evenly.
8. Top chicken with buffalo wing sauce.
9. Put the ranch dressing on top of sauce.
10. Sprinkle grated cheese.
11. On top of cheese, spread the diced scallions.
12. **Without cover, bake for 20 minutes at 350°F or up to point cheese is melted.**
13. Serve warm with blue corn chips.

8. Potato Soup Infused With Bacon And Chives

Ingredients:

- Fresh chopped chives, for garnish
- 2 tbsp olive oil
- Salt and pepper, to taste
- 4 medium size potatoes -yukon gold or red skin, peeled and chopped into bite size chunks
- ½ cup Pepper Jack cheese, grated (can sub in grated cheddar)-reduced fat can work too
- 3 fresh thyme sprigs
- ½ cup buttermilk or (FODMAPers use lactose free milk)
- 4 cups of chicken broth (FODMAPers use homemade broth)
- Bacon, 1 slice per person, cooked and crumbled
- ½ cup sliced, washed leeks (white part or green part) or chives
- Bread bowl if you choose (you may choose the right gluten free roll)

Instructions

1. In a medium stock pot for sauce, saute oil and chives for about 1 minute in medium heat.
2. Put in thyme, potatoes, and broth and bring to a boil. Have medium-low heat, then simmer.
3. Cook potatoes for around 40 minutes or until tender. Remove soup from heat and allow to cool down for around 15 minutes.
4. Put soup slowly in blender and blend with consistent smoothness.
5. Combine buttermilk and cheese with the soup in a stock pot and cook just to warm the soup and have cheese melted.
6. Flavor with pepper and salt.
7. Serve in bowl for soup or bread (use gluten free).
8. Add garnishings of chives and bacon.

9. Macaroni & Cheese Recipe

Ingredients:

- ½ tsp gluten free asafoetida powder (**garlic & onion substitute**)
- 1 tsp salt
- ¾ cup **rice milk** (or any other lactose free milk)
- 1 tbsp gluten free flour
- 1 cup shredded cheese (You may use ½ cup cheddar and ½ cup parmesan.)
- 1 tbsp lactose free butter
- 1 teaspoon pepper
- 8 oz gluten free macaroni or pasta

Instructions:

1. Over high heat, cook pasta in a large saucepan.
2. With medium heat, heat milk in small saucepan as pasta is cooked.
3. Add butter to milk.
4. Turn off heat when butter is melted and then mix with salt, pepper, and gluten free flour.
5. Add the cheese.
6. Drain when pasta is cooked instead of rinsing with cold water.
7. Put together the cheese and pasta mixture.

10. Stir Fry Sesame Chicken Ala Asia

Ingredients:

- 2-3 cups of veggies of your choice (Recommended are Swiss chard, summer squash, and mini eggplant.)
- ¾ lb thinly sliced boneless skinless chicken breast
- 1 tbsp minced ginger
- 1 tbsp sesame oil
- 1 tbsp sesame seeds (You may use a mixture of black seeds and traditional seeds.)
- 2 tbsp soy sauce
- **1 tbsp olive oil**

Instructions:

1. Combine sesame oil, minced ginger, and soy sauce in medium size glass bowl.
2. Immerse chicken in marinade and keep in the refrigerator for 15 minutes to an hour, turning chicken over for even coverage until ready to cook.
3. Cook chicken on non-stick skillet over medium heat until chicken is browned and thoroughly cooked through. Transfer chicken to plate.
4. Pour 1 tbsp oil in the same skillet and sauté vegetables until al dente.
5. Put back chicken. Microwave brown rice at the same time.

Put rice into skillet and stir to blend using a little bit of soy sauce. Serve immediately.

11. Potato Soup

Ingredients:

- ½ cup shredded parmesan cheese
- 2 tsp pepper
- 2 32-oz cans of chicken broth
- 1 tsp dried oregano
- ¼ cup fresh chives, diced
- Bacon, cooked and crumbled as desired (optional)
- 2 tbsp fresh parsley, diced
- 3 tsp Kosher salt
- 1 bunch of green onions, diced (green part only)
- 2 tsp gluten free asafoetida powder (garlic & onion replacement)
- 1 tsp dried basil
- 6-8 large potatoes, peeled & cut into 1-inch squares
- 3 tbsp garlic infused olive oil
- ½ cup shredded parmesan cheese
- ½ cup rice milk (or any other lactose free milk), warmed

Instructions:

1. In a large pot, place green onions, potatoes, carrots, broth, and chives.
2. Let mixture come to a boil and stir often.
3. Put in basil, pepper, parsley, oregano, olive oil, salt, and asafoetida powder.
4. Decrease heat and cook for 30-40 minutes or as potatoes become tender with occasional stirring.
5. When softened remove potatoes from heat and mash to blend well.
6. Mix with parmesan cheese and milk making sure to stir to blend mixture adequately.
7. If to serve at once add bacon and stir.
8. Sprinkle chives and parmesan cheese.
9. Place in microwavable plastic containers sized 2-3 cups and store in a freezer.

12. Zucchini Cake

Ingredients:

- ¼ tsp almond extract
- 1 medium zucchini, grated (about 2 cups)
- 1/3 cup sliced almonds
- ¼ cup oil (You can use melted coconut oil)
- ½ tsp baking soda
- 2 large eggs, whisked
- ½ tsp almond extract
- ¼ cup granulated sugar
- 1 tsp vanilla extract
- 1/3 cup unsweetened coconut* optional
- 1 ½ cup unbleached all-purpose or whole-wheat pastry flour
- 2 tbsp brown sugar
- ½ tsp baking powder
- 4 ounce plain low fat Greek yogurt (FODMAP followers use lactose free plain yogurt if you want, though the amount of lactose per serving is quite low with the Greek yogurt.)

FOR GLAZE:

- ½ cup confectioner's sugar
- 4 tbsp melted butter
- **2 tsp + water**

Instructions:

1. Prepare oven by preheating in 350°F.
2. Lightly oil a square 8x8 pan.
3. Stir to blend a mixture of yogurt, melted butter, zucchini, oil, and eggs in medium bowl.
4. Add and blend in extracts, coconut, and sugars.
5. Gradually add and thoroughly blend in baking powder, baking soda, and flour.
6. Include almonds this time.
7. Bake the entire mixture into the prepared pan for about 30 minutes.

For a yummy-looking glaze, combine confectioner's almond extract, water, and sugar in a bowl. Transform it to a soup with thick consistency by whisking adding water as necessary. Sprinkle over cake.

13. Roasted Shrimp In Lemon Parsley

Ingredients:

- ¼ cup shredded parmesan cheese
- 1 lb extra large shrimp (peeled and de-veined)
- ½ tsp crushed red pepper flakes
- 2 tbsp lemon juice
- 2 tbsp garlic infused oil
- **¼ freshly chopped parsley**
- sea salt and pepper, to taste

Instructions:

1. Prepare oven by preheating to 400°F.
2. Put a little oil on cookie sheet.
3. Gently dry shrimp with paper towel and spread in cookie sheet evenly.
4. Stir together oil, crushed red pepper, lemon, sea salt and pepper to taste in small bowl and sprinkle evenly over shrimp.
5. For 6-8 minutes roast the shrimp until fully cooked and opaque.

   Take out shrimp from oven and sprinkle with fresh parsley and shredded parmesan cheese.

14. Pineapple Salsa

Ingredients: Serves about 6

- 1 tbsp chopped parsley or cilantro
- Top 1 tbsp salsa on top of grilled fresh corn tortilla topped with 1/4 cup grated cheddar cheese, beef or chicken strips, and 5 grilled shrimp
- 1 tbsp olive oil
- 1 tsp lime zest
- 1 tbsp fresh lime juice
- 1 medium jalapeño, deseeded and diced {optional}
- ¼ cup green bell pepper, deseeded, and diced
- ½ cup cherry tomatoes, diced in quarters
- 1 cup fresh diced fresh pineapple
- **Salt and pepper, to taste**

Instructions:

1. Combine the ingredients and include fresh herbs prior to serving.
2. Can be prepared and placed in refrigerator a day ahead.

15. Teriyaki Chicken Meatballs

Ingredients: Serves 4-6

- Garnish: chopped green part of scallion, toasted sesame seeds
- 1 ½ lb ground chicken breast
- ½ cup diced red bell pepper
- 1 egg
- 1 tbsp fresh minced ginger
- 2 scallions, chopped (green part only, FODMAPers)--extra for garnish
- ½ cup water
- ½ tbsp toasted sesame oil
- 2 tbsp light brown sugar
- ½ cup reduced sodium soy sauce
- ½ tbsp toasted sesame oil
- 1 tbsp reduced sodium soy sauce (Use gluten free if following gluten free diet)
- ¼ cup diced pineapple
- 1 tbsp fresh minced ginger
- 1 tbsp cornstarch
- 1/3 cup brown rice bread crumbs
- **Cooked rice, if desired**

   Instructions:

1. Prepare oven by preheating to 350°F.
2. Lightly oil cookie sheet.
3. Blend together chicken, sesame oil, egg, scallions, crumbs, soy sauce, ginger in medium bowl.
4. Make around 30 meatballs out of mixture and place in cookie sheet.
5. Baking the meatballs should take some 20 minutes.
6. Combine and stir to blend all ingredients for sauce excluding cornstarch in large skillet, in average heat.
7. Add the meatballs making sure they immerse in the sauce. Let it cook for around 4 minutes.

8. Whisk together cornstarch and 2 tbsp of water in small bowl.
9. Combine cornstarch mixture with meatballs mixture for a gravy consistency in sauce.

Serve with rice, if wanted, and put toasted seeds of sesame and few slices of scallion over top of meatballs.

16. Poached Salmon And Vege Risotto

Ingredients: serves 4-6
500g salmon fillets, skin on or off

Stock
10 peppercorns
1 leek
2 bay leaves
5 parsley stalks
1 stick celery
2 tbsp lemon juice, optional
1 teaspoon salt
1 carrot
1.7 l water

Risotto

2 cups (425g) risotto rice
1 cup (40g) finely grated parmesan cheese
1 leek
finely grated zest of 1 lemon

1 tbsp baby capers, or chop if a little big
¼ cup (60ml) dry white wine, optional
1 tsp each butter and garlic infused oil
For the stock, chop off the leek's green top and wash with other vegetables. Roughly chop everything and combine with bay leaves, salt, pepper, and water in a pot. Bring to a boil then cover the pot, lower the heat letting it simmer for 30 minutes. Lower the heat and place salmon in the stock with pot covered for 8-10 minutes until cooked. Transfer salmon into a plate and remove the skin, then cut the fillet in bite-sized flakes. Place

stock in saucepan to drain and discard the vegetables. Maintain low heat.

For the risotto, chop off again the green top from second leek. Cut the leaves in half then shred. Over low heat, combine the leek with butter and oil and saute for 8-10 minutes without browning. Lower heat to medium and include rice stirring for one more minute. Pour in wine and stir until absorbed. One more cup stock and stir until absorbed. Keep adding stock until rice is soft enough. Combine the flaked salmon, lemon zest, parmesan, and capers and fold.

What Is This So Called Fodmap Diet?

This may be your first time of hearing the term FODMAP, so what is it exactly? Is it another diet craze in the market out to rob you of your hard earned cash? I will leave that decision to you once you get to know FODMAP better.

FODMAP stands for **F**ermentable **O**ligo-**D**i-**M**onosaccharides and **P**olyols. FODMAP are mainly carbohydrate rich foods that are osmotic. If you refresh yourself with your chemistry, osmosis is a process by which water is pulled from a low gradient to a higher gradient. In the gut, FODMAPs can pull water into the intestinal tract. These foods are not easily absorbed or digested well and when eaten in excess can be acted upon by bacteria through fermentation.

People who are sensitive to FODMAP can experience cramping, bloating, gas, constipation or diarrhea. That's why a LOW FODMAP diet is being promoted in order to avoid experiencing these symptoms.

The Low FODMAP diet is highly recommended for people who are suffering from Irritable Bowel Syndrome (IBS). This diet is also recommended for other digestive problems like inflammatory bowel disease or other digestive problems with similar presenting symptoms.

FODMAP Foods

To easily identify FODMAP foods, here is a quick and generalized description of them:

- Polyols – these would pertain to sweeteners that contain xylitol, sorbitol, mannitol, and isomalt; stone fruits like plums, peaches, nectarines, cherries, apricots, avocadoes and others.

- Galactans – these are legume like soybeans, lentils, beans and others
- Lactose – foods that contain dairy
- Fructose – this is sugars found in fruits, high fructose corn syrup (HFCS), honey and others.

Your FODMAP Chart

Food Group	High FODMAPs Food (Foods to AVOID)	Low FODMAPs
Condiments and Seasonings	artificial sweeteners, tomato paste, onion powder/salt, onions, molasses, hummus, honey, garlic powder/salt, garlic, agave, salad dressing or sauce with HFCS, (salsa, relish, pickle, jelly, jam, and chutney—that contain HFCS)	Vinegar, soy sauce, sugar, seeds *sunflower, sesame, pumpkin, flax, and chia), salt, pesto, pepper, olives, spring onion green part, mayonnaise, margarine, mustard, most spices and herbs, homemade broth, cooking oils, chives, butter, garli/onion infused oil, the following without HFCS: maple syrup, salad dressing, sauces, salsa, relish, pickle, jelly, jam.
Drinks	Tea, coffee, fruit and vegetable smoothies made from allowed foods (limit to ½ cup	Those made with HFCS, fortified wines like port or sherry.

166

	at a time).	
Desserts	Made from allowed foods	Foods made with HFCS
Vegetables	Sugar snap peas, mushrooms, cauliflower, and artichokes	zucchini, water chestnuts, turnips, tomatoes, squash, spinach, seaweed, rutabaga, radishes, potatoes, pumpkin, parsnips, lettuce, kale, green beans, eggplant, cucumbers, cabbage, carrots, bok choy, bell peppers, bamboo shoots, bean sprouts, alfalfa sprouts.
Fruits	watermelon, prunes, persimmon, plums, pears, peaches, papaya, nectarines, mango, guava, figs, dried fruits, dates, canned fruit, boysenberries, blackberries, apricots, applesauce, apples	tangerine, strawberries, rhubarb, raspberries, pineapple, passion fruit, orange, mandarin, lime, lemon, kiwi, honeydew, grapes, cranberries, cantaloupe, blueberries, bananas.
Grains	inulin, chicory root, gluten free or spelt grains made with foods to limit, foods made with rye/barley or wheat as the major ingredient.	foods that are made from spelt or gluten free grains like tapioca, rice, quinoa, potato, oats and corn; rice bran, rice, quinoa, popcorn, oat bran,

		oatmeal, waffles, tortillas, pretzels, pastas, pancakes, noodles, crackers, chips, cereals, breads, biscuits, bagels.
Meat, non-dairy alternatives	soy milk from soybeans, soybeans, pistachios, miso, lentils, bulgur, black eyed peas, beans, cashews.	tofu, tempeh, nut butters, nuts (like pine, pecan, peanut, macadamia, walnut), milk alternatives (soymilk from soy protein, rice, coconut, almond)
Dairy	High lactose dairy: sour cream, soft cheeses (ricotta, cottage, etc.), Milk (condensed, evaporated, sheep's, goat's, cow's), ice cream, custard, cheesy or creamy sauces, chocolate and buttermilk.	Lactose free or low lactose dairy: whipped cream, Greek yogurt, sherbet soft cheeses (mozzarella, feta, brie, etc.), hard cheeses (Swiss, parmesan, Colby, cheddar, etc.), half and half, cream cheese
Fish, poultry, meat and eggs	Foods made with HFCS or foods to limit	turkey, shellfish, pork, lamb, fish, eggs, deli slices, chicken and beef

Moderate FODMAPs or Foods to Limit

These foods are considered to be moderate FODMAPs so eat in moderation. If you experience symptoms from eating any of these foods, then avoid. Also, when consuming foods that are moderate FODMAPs follow the recommended serving sizes.

Fruits	Vegetables	Nuts
<10 dried banana chips	<1/2 cup sweet potato	<10 hazelnuts
<1/4 cup shredded coconut	½ corn cob	<10 almonds
½ pomegranate	<10 pods snow peas	
<3 rambutan	3 okra pods	
<5 lychee	<1/2 cup green peas	
<10 longan	1 celery stick	
½ grapefruit (medium)	< 1 cup cabbage (savoy)	
<3 cherries	<1/4 cup butternut pumpkin	
¼ avocado	<1/2 cup brussels sprouts	
	<1/2 cup broccoli	
	4 beet slices	
	<3 asparagus spears	
	¼ cup artichoke hearts	

Low FODMAP Diet Tips

Here is a list of tips to help you follow the Low FODMAP diet easily and help you control your IBS problems:

- If you experience constipation while on a low FODMAP diet, you should drink more water and include high fiber but low FODMAP foods like oatmeal to help ease and prevent constipation.
- When it comes to eating low FODMAP veggies and fruits plus low lactose dairy, keep it to ½ cup per meal—in total. If ever you experience problems after eating these types of food, it

could be due to eating large amounts of FODMAPs all at once.

- It is recommended that you buy gluten free grains that do not contain rye, barley or wheat. But, you can eat grains with gluten because in this diet you are concerned with FODMAPs rather than gluten.

- When buying food, learn to read food labels and identify low FODMAP foods. Remember that high FODMAP foods are to be avoided especially those containing soy, wheat, inulin, honey and HFCS.

- Before going on this diet, we highly recommend that you collect low FODMAP recipes first, create a grocery list and go on a grocery shopping with enough time to spare on reading food labels. Once you are done, you can begin the diet and stick to it for six weeks.

- Once the FODMAP diet trial is over, one at a time add the high FODMAP foods into your diet in little amounts. This way, you can pinpoint which foods will trigger your symptoms and thereby avoid these foods or limit intake if possible.

- Knowing that the FODMAP diet can be a bit restrictive when it comes to creating your food, researchers have found that a key factor in helping people stick to the diet is to factor food preference and lifestyle behaviors. Do not prepare foods just because it is Low FODMAP, also ensure that you like it and it tastes good. Balance those adventure times when you create dishes out of the blue and sticking to your old time favorites.

- Plan ahead is always the key for a successful FODMAP diet. Since there are quite a lot of foods that are to be avoided, chances are with a weekly planned meal and planned grocery shopping, you can stick better to your Low FODMAP diet.

- Have safe snacks on hand so that you won't be encouraged to eat whatever's available just to satisfy your hunger. Here's a quick list of safe snacks that you can keep on hand in your pantry or ref:

- One celery stick filled with peanut butter
- One banana with a handful of almonds
- Swiss cheese and Blue diamond almond nut thins
- Two rice cakes with a layer of peanut butter
- Lactose free yogurt with a cup of blueberries
- Mozzarella cheese stick and Glutino pretzels
- Have colorful fruits low in FODMAPs in your ref like: kiwi, oranges, pineapple, cantaloupe, grapes, blueberries, bananas and strawberries.

Low Fodmap Diet Recipes

Fodmap Breakfast Recipes

Eggs Florentine

Servings per Recipe: 4
Ingredients:

4 slices ciabatta sourdough, toasted
4 fresh eggs, at room temperature
Dash of white vinegar
2 bunches English spinach, trimmed, washed and dried
2 tbsps butter
8 thin bacon rashers
Hollandaise Ingredients:

2 tsps lemon juice
1 cup butter unsalted and melted
2 egg yolks
1 shallot, finely chopped
6 black peppercorns
¼ cup white wine vinegar
Directions:

1) Make the hollandaise sauce by mixing on low heat in a small saucepan the shallot, peppercorns and vinegar. Simmer uncovered until mixture is reduced to 2 tsps around 3 to 5 minutes. Remove from fire and strain into a heat proof bowl.

2)   Add egg yolks and whisk mixture placed inside a pan with simmering hot water. Add slowly butter while whisking continuously. Continue heating and whisking until creamy. Turn off fire, season with pepper and salt to taste. Whisk in lemon juice and set aside.

3)On high fire place a nonstick fry pan and cook bacon until crisped. Transfer to a plate.

4)   On same pan, discard bacon oil and heat butter. Cook spinach until wilted around 3 to 4 minutes and season to taste with pepper and salt.

5)   In a fry pan filled halfway with water, bring to a boil. Lower fire and poach 1 egg until cooked to desired doneness. With a slotted spoon, remove egg and cook remaining eggs the same way, one at a time.

6)To assemble, place toast on 4 serving plates. Layer with spinach, bacon, poached eggs and drizzle with hollandaise sauce. Serve and enjoy.

Ham And Spinach Frittata

Servings per Recipe: 4
Ingredients:

9 oz cherry tomatoes, halved
6 eggs
Pepper and salt to taste
2 oz ham, chopped
1 bunch English spinach, trimmed and shredded
Directions:

1) In a big bowl, whisk eggs, pepper and salt to taste.

2)   Grease an 8 x 8 inch baking dish and preheat oven to 375oF.

3)On dish make 4 layers of spinach and ham.

4)   Pour egg mixture into dish.

5)   Top with tomato halves with the cut side up.

6)Pop in the oven and bake until set around 35 to 40 minutes.

7)Remove from oven, let it stand for 10 minutes, slice equally and serve.

Oatmeal With Pecans And Cinnamon

Servings per Recipe: 4

Ingredients:

Pinch of salt
1 tbsp ground flax seeds
2 tbsps cacao nibs
4 tbsps raisins
1 ½ tsp cinnamon
¼ cup pecans
1 tsp pure vanilla extract
2 cups purified water
2 cups rice milk
1 cup gluten free steel cut oats
Directions:

1) On high fire, place a medium pot and boil rice milk and water.

2)   Once boiling, add oats and cook around 20 minutes or until soft.

3)Decrease fire to low and add remaining ingredients.

4)   Continue cooking for another two minutes.

5)   Remove from fire and equally place oatmeal on to 4 bowls.

6)Serve and enjoy while warm.

Rice, Bacon And Chicken Bake

Servings per Recipe: 4
Ingredients:

¼ cup coriander leaves
2 cups Campbell's real stock chicken
1 small lemon, rind grated and juiced
1 tsp ground turmeric
2 garlic cloves, crushed
6 green onions, sliced thinly
1 cup SunRice white long grain rice
2 tbsps olive oil
8 skinless chicken thigh fillets
8 rashers middle bacon, rind removed, divided
Directions:

1) Grease a 9 x 9 casserole dish and preheat oven to 350oF.

2) Slice in half 4 pieces of bacon rashers lengthwise and wrap one slice around per chicken thigh fillet and secure with a toothpick. Minced the remaining 4 pieces of bacon rashers.

3)On medium high fire, place a fry pan and heat oil. In batches, pan fry chicken until bacon is lightly browned around 2 minutes per side. Transfer to a plate and cook remaining chicken pieces same way.

4) On same and empty fry pan, add minced bacon and rice. Cook on low fire for a minute while stirring. Add pepper, salt, stock, lemon rind, turmeric, garlic and onions. Stir fry for a minute.

5) Place rice on bottom of greased dish. Add chicken thighs on top and press down gently on rice.

6)Cover dish with foil and pop into the oven. Bake until chicken is cooked through and rice is tender, around 50 minutes.

7)Remove from oven; let it stand for ten minutes.

8)   Remove toothpicks, sprinkle with coriander leaves and drizzle with lemon juice before serving.

Millet Porridge

Servings per Recipe: 4
Ingredients:

¼ tsp sea salt
¼ tsp almond extract
2 tbsps ground flax seeds
2 tbsps coconut flakes
2 tbsps cinnamon
2 tbsp carob powder
1 tsp dairy free vegan butter
1 tsp maple syrup
½ cup raw almonds
1 cup almond milk
1 cup uncooked millet
Directions:

1) Grease a baking sheet and preheat oven to 375oF.

2)   According to package instructions, cook millet.

3)While cooking, mix well carob powder, butter, maple syrup and almonds in a large bowl.

4)   Spread mixture on prepared sheet and pop in the oven. Bake until toasted around 30 minutes. Remove from oven and set aside.

5)   Equally divide into 4 bowls the cooked millet. Top with sea salt, almond extract, flax seeds, coconut flakes, toasted almonds and almond milk.

6)Serve and enjoy.

Fodmap Lunch Recipes

Fodmap Free Seafood Chowder

Servings per Recipe: 6
Ingredients:

Crusty French bread
2 tbsps chopped fresh parsley
2 tbsps chopped fresh chives
Sea salt
200 ml thickened cream
500g gourmet marinara mix
2 corn cobs
4 cups Campbell's real stock chicken
3 (750g) potatoes, peeled, roughly chopped
1 stick celery, finely chopped
1 medium carrot, finely chopped
Directions:

1) On high fire, place a large sauce pan and bring to a boil stock, potatoes, celery, and carrot. Once boiling, reduce fire to a simmer and cook until tender, around 10 minutes.

2) Turn off fire, stir to cool for 10 minutes, transfer to a blender and puree until smooth.

3)Pour pureed mixture back to pan and continue cooking on medium low fire.

4) Remove kernels from corn cobs and add to soup. Cook until tender around 10 minutes.

5) Add cream and marinara mix.

6)Continue cooking and stirring until chowder is cooked though.

7)Season to taste. Add parsley and chives.

8) Divide equally into 4 bowls and serve while hot.

Celery And Cos Salad

Servings per Recipe: 10
Ingredients:

1 cup pecan nuts, toasted, chopped
5 sticks celery, sliced diagonally
1 cos lettuce, roughly torn
Lemon Dressing Ingredients:

1 ½ tsps brown sugar
¼ cup lemon juice
1/3 cup olive oil
Directions:

1) To make the dressing, in a lidded jar, mix all ingredients and season with pepper and salt to taste. Cover tightly with lid and vigorously shake to mix.

2)   In a salad bowl, mix half the nuts, celery and lettuce.

3)Drizzle dressing and toss to mix.

4)   Garnish with remaining nuts, serve and enjoy.

Dijon Mustard Cream Sauce With Chicken

Servings per Recipe: 4
Ingredients:

Fresh parsley or cilantro
Pepper and salt to taste
¾ cup FODMAP free sour cream
1 tsp dried thyme
½ cup Dijon mustard
Olive oil
8 pcs of chicken or 4 pieces chicken breast
Directions:

1) Grease a shallow baking pan with olive oil and preheat oven to 400oF.

2) In a medium bowl, mix well sour cream, thyme and mustard. Divide mustard sauce in two bowls.

3)Coat chicken using 1 bowl of mustard mixture and place on prepped baking dish.

4) Cover dish with foil tightly and pop in the oven until chicken is cooked around 50 to 60 minutes.

5) Meanwhile, season remaining mustard mixture with pepper and salt to taste.

6)Once chicken is cooked, pour chicken drippings into remaining mustard mixture and mix well.

7)To serve, pour seasoned mustard mixture over chicken and enjoy.

Low Fodmap Tacos

Servings per Recipe: 4 to 6

Ingredients:

12 corn tortillas
Taco seasoning
½ cup water
1 can organic tomato sauce (ensure that it contains no garlic and
    onion)
1 red bell pepper, chopped (optional)
2 tbsps chopped chives
1 lb ground beef
1 head Cos lettuce, shredded
3 cups shredded Mexican cheese
Taco Seasoning Ingredients:

1 tsp black pepper
1 tsp salt
1 ½ tsps ground cumin
½ tsp paprika
¼ tsp dried oregano
¼ tsp crushed red pepper flakes
1 tbsp chili powder
Directions:

1) To make taco seasoning, mix well all ingredients in a bowl and
put aside.

2) To make taco, on medium fire place a large nonstick
saucepan and stir fry bell pepper, chives and beef. Cook beef
until browned and discard fat.

3)Meanwhile, in an oven, toast corn tortillas until heated
through.

4) Then add water, tomato sauce and seasonings into
saucepan and simmer for 20 minutes on low fire.

5) To assemble, evenly divide meat mixture into twelve and place onto taco shells, topped by shredded lettuce, diced tomatoes, and cheese.

6)Serve and enjoy.

Turkey Meatballs Fodmap Free

Servings per Recipe: 34 Meatballs
Ingredients:

2 eggs slightly beaten
1 tsp coarse ground pepper
2 tsps salt
1 tbsp sage
1 tbsp dried chives
1 tbsp dried oregano
8 slices gluten free bread
2 lbs ground turkey

Directions:

1) Grease a broiler rack and preheat broiler.

2)   In a large mixing bowl, place ground turkey.

3)Place bread under running water, and squeeze out excess moisture and crumble bread into bowl.

4)   Add remaining ingredients into bowl and mix well with hands until mixture is thoroughly incorporated.

5)   Form balls out of mixture as big as 1.5-inch in diameter and place on to prepped broiler rack.

6)Once all meat is formed into balls, pop broiler into oven and broil for 8 minutes.

7)Remove pan from oven and turnover meatballs. Return to oven and cook for another 8 minutes.

8)   Remove from oven and let it stand for 8 minutes before serving.

Fodmap Snack Recipes

Fodmap Free Nut Biscuits

Servings per Recipe: 22 biscuits

Ingredients:

1 cup unsalted mixed nuts with sultanas, chopped roughly
1 cup rice flour
2 tbsps natural yogurt
1 tsp vanilla extract
1 large egg, lightly beaten
½ firmly packed cup brown sugar
125 g butter, softened

Directions:

1) Grease 2 baking sheets with cooking spray and preheat oven to 350oF.

2)   In a mixing bowl, beat sugar and butter until light and fluffy.

3)Add vanilla and egg. Mix well.

4)   Fold nut mix, flour and yoghurt.

5)   With a measuring tablespoon, get a slightly rounded dough of the mixture, drop onto prepped baking sheet and flatten into circular biscuits. Repeat until all mixture is used up.

6)Pop into the oven and bake until lightly browned around 12 minutes.

7)Serve and enjoy. Biscuits can be stored for 3 days in a tightly lidded container.

Zucchini Bread

Servings per Recipe: 6 to 8
Ingredients:

½ cup sunflower seeds
¼ tsp fresh lemon zest
¼ tsp all spice
1 ½ tbsp ground cinnamon
½ cup coconut flour
1 tsp gluten free baking powder
½ tsp baking soda
¼ tsp Himalayan sea salt
½ cup organic coconut oil, melted
1 cup coconut sugar
1 ½ tbsp almond extract
2 cups ripe zucchini, shredded
3 large eggs
Directions:

1) Grease a bread pan and preheat oven to 350oF.

2)   Beat eggs until fluffy in a mixing bowl.

3)Add coconut sugar, almond extract and zucchini. Mix well.

4)   While whisking continuously, add coconut oil slowly.

5)   In a separate bowl, sift coconut flour and discard lumps. Add sunflower seeds, lemon zest, all spice, cinnamon, coconut flour, almond flour, baking powder, baking soda and salt. Mix well to combine.

6)Slowly stir in dry ingredients into wet ingredients. Mix until no lumps are seen.

7)Pour batter into prepared bread pan, pop into the oven and bake until set around 50 to 60 minutes.

8)   Remove from oven and let it cook for 15 minutes, slice and serve while warm.

Pumpkin Seeds, Coconut Yogurt On Cherry Parfait

Servings per Recipe: 4
Ingredients:

2 tbsps unsweetened coconut flakes
4 tbsps shelled pumpkin seeds or pepitas
1 cup gluten free granola
24 fresh cherries cut in half
½ tsp cinnamon powder
3 tbsps maple syrup
2 cups coconut milk yogurt
Directions:

1) Mix well cinnamon honey and yogurt in a small bowl.

2)   In parfait glasses, layer yogurt mixture, granola and cherries.

3)Top with coconut flakes and pumpkin seeds.

4)   Place in the freezer for 30 minutes and serve chilled.

Almond Vegan Fodmap Free Cookies

Servings per Recipe: 12
Ingredients:

¼ cup cacao nibs
¼ cup crushed almonds
½ tsp cocoa powder
½ cup coconut sugar
¼ tsp sea salt
1 cup quinoa flakes
1 cup cooked quinoa
1 tsp almond extract
3 large ripe bananas, peeled and mashed
1 tsp almond butter
Directions:

1) Grease a baking sheet and preheat oven to 375oF.

2) Mix well coconut sugar, almond extract, bananas and almond butter in a big mixing bowl.

3)Add sea salt, quinoa flakes, and cooked quinoa. Thoroughly mix.

4) Add cacao nibs, crushed almonds and cocoa powder. Blend well.

5) Place golf ball sizes of the dough mixture on to the prepared baking sheet. Ensure that batter is at least 1-inch apart. Continue rolling the dough until mixture is used up.

6)Place baking sheet in preheated oven and bake until golden brown around 20 to 25 minutes.

7)Once cooked, remove cookies from oven and transfer to a wire rack. Let it cool for ten minutes before serving.

8) Cookies can be stored in tightly lidded containers for up to 3 days.